# Essential Practices in Hospice and Palliative Medicine

Fifth Edition

# Essential Practices in Hospice and Palliative Medicine
Fifth Edition

## UNIPAC 3
# PAIN ASSESSMENT AND MANAGEMENT

**Mellar P. Davis, MD FCCP FAAHPM**
Geisinger Medical Center
Danville, PA

**Shalini Dalal, MD**
University of Texas MD Anderson Cancer Center
Houston, TX

**Harold Goforth, MD**
The Cleveland Clinic
Cleveland, OH

**Mary Lynn McPherson, PharmD MA MDE BCPS CPE**
University of Maryland School of Pharmacy
Baltimore, MD

**Eric Roeland, MD FAAHPM**
UC San Diego Moores Cancer Center
La Jolla, CA

**Paul A. Sloan, MD**
University of Kentucky
Lexington, KY

*Reviewed by*
**Perry G. Fine, MD**
University of Utah
Salt Lake City, UT

*Edited by*
**Joseph W. Shega, MD**
Vitas Healthcare
Miami, FL

**Miguel A. Paniagua, MD FACP**
University of Pennsylvania
Philadelphia, PA

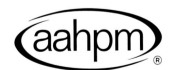

AMERICAN ACADEMY OF
HOSPICE AND PALLIATIVE MEDICINE

8735 W. Higgins Rd., Ste. 300
Chicago, IL 60631
aahpm.org | PalliativeDoctors.org

The information presented and opinions expressed herein are those of the editors and authors and do not necessarily represent the views of the American Academy of Hospice and Palliative Medicine. Any recommendations made by the editors and authors must be weighed against the healthcare provider's own clinical judgment, based on but not limited to such factors as the patient's condition, benefits versus risks of suggested treatment, and comparison with recommendations of pharmaceutical compendia and other medical and palliative care authorities.

Some discussions of pharmacological treatments in *Essential Practices in Hospice and Palliative Medicine* may describe off-label uses of drugs commonly used by hospice and palliative medicine providers. "Good medical practice and the best interests of the patient require that physicians use legally available drugs, biologics, and devices according to their best knowledge and judgment. If physicians use a product for an indication not in the approved labeling, they have the responsibility to be well informed about the product, to base its use on firm scientific rationale and on sound medical evidence, and to maintain records of the product's use and effects. Use of a marketed product in this manner *when the intent is the 'practice of medicine'* does not require the submission of an Investigational New Drug Application (IND), Investigational Device Exemption (IDE), or review by an Institutional Review Board (IRB). However, the institution at which the product will be used may, under its own authority, require IRB review or other institutional oversight" (US Food and Drug Administration, https://www.fda.gov/RegulatoryInformation/Guidances/ucm126486.htm. Updated January 25, 2016. Accessed May 17, 2017).

Published in the United States by the American Academy of Hospice and Palliative Medicine, 8735 W. Higgins Rd., Ste. 300, Chicago, IL 60631.

## AAHPM Education Staff

Julie Bruno, Director, Education and Learning
Kemi Ani, Manager, Education and Learning
Angie Forbes, Manager, Education and Learning
Angie Tryfonopoulos, Coordinator, Education and
   Learning

## AAHPM Editorial Staff

Jerrod Liveoak, Senior Editorial Manager
Bryan O'Donnell, Managing Editor
Andie Bernard, Assistant Editor
Tim Utesch, Graphic Designer
Jean Iversen, Copy Editor

ISBN 978-1-889296-23-4

# Contents

# Tables

# Figures

# Acknowledgments

AAHPM is deeply grateful to all who have participated in the development of this component of the *Essential Practices in Hospice and Palliative Medicine* self-study program. The expertise of the editors, contributors, and reviewers involved in the current and previous editions of the *Essentials* series has ensured the value of its content to our field.

AAHPM extends special thanks to the authors of previous editions of this volume, Sharon M. Weinstein, MD FAAHPM, Russell K. Portenoy, MD, Sarah E. Harrington, MD, Andrea Bial, MD, Stacie Levine, MD, C. Porter Storey, Jr., MD FACP FAAHPM, and Carol F. Knight, EdM; the authors of the *UNIPAC 3 amplifire* online learning module, Mellar P. Davis, MD FCCP FAAHPM, and Paul A. Sloan, MD; the pharmacist reviewer for this edition of the *Essentials* series, Jennifer Pruskowski, Pharm D; and the many professionals who volunteered their time and expertise to review the content and test this program in the field—Joseph Rotella, MD MBA HMDC FAAHPM, C. Porter Storey, Jr., MD FACP FAAHPM, Joseph W. Shega, MD, Stacie Levine, MD, Judith A. Paice, PhD RN, Linda King, MD, Perry G. Fine, MD, John W. Finn, MD FAAHPM, Gerald H. Holman, MD FAAFP, Eli N. Perencevich, DO, and Julia L. Smith, MD.

*Essentials in Hospice and Palliative Medicine* was originally published in 1998 in six volumes as the *UNIPAC* self-study program. The first four editions of this series, which saw the introduction of three new volumes, were created under the leadership of C. Porter Storey, Jr., MD FACP FAAHPM, who served as author and editor. AAHPM is proud to acknowledge Dr. Storey's commitment to and leadership of this expansive and critical resource. The Academy's gratitude for his innumerable contributions cannot be overstated.

## Continuing Medical Education

Continuing medical education credits are available, and Maintenance of Certification credits may be available, to users who complete the *amplifire* online learning module that has been created for each volume of *Essential Practices in Hospice and Palliative Medicine*, available for purchase from aahpm.org.

# The Persistent Problem of Pain

People with life-threatening or life-limiting illnesses frequently experience pain, and many have multiple comorbidities that are also painful. Therapeutic advancements have changed the trajectories of many diseases, but extended survival may be complicated by persistent pain and other symptoms. For instance, for patients with advanced cancer, targeted anticancer therapies, immunotherapy, and newer chemotherapies may increase the likelihood of a cure or prolonged survival but with an attendant life-altering burden of symptoms arising from the cumulative effects of disease progression and adverse effects of treatment.[1]

A patient's experience of pain is influenced by psychosocial and spiritual factors as well as biological mechanisms. Distress in any of these dimensions can affect perception of the intensity, source, and meaning of the pain and its interference with quality of life (QOL). The best practice in pain management is an integrated approach that is multidisciplinary, affordable, available, patient centered, and compassionate. An empathetic, patient-centered approach to pain management is as important to the success of relieving the suffering caused by pain as any medications that may be prescribed.[2]

A steady stream of progress in basic science pain research since the mid 2000s has paved the way for development of novel pain treatments, but, for now, the pharmacological management of pain is limited to a few classes of analgesics with significant side effects and a narrow therapeutic index. As more physicians have prescribed opioids for all sorts of pain syndromes, there has been an increase in opioid overdose deaths that is now recognized as a public health crisis. Well-intentioned campaigns to improve pain management for patients with cancer and other serious illnesses may have contributed to inappropriate prescribing. For example, some authors have linked the "pain as the fifth vital sign" campaign to an overreliance on opioids by novice prescribers, resulting in increased hospital adverse events.[3-5]

When considering prescribing opioids for pain, it can be a challenge to find the right balance between relieving suffering and preventing harm, and there are no simple shortcuts. It is important to consider not only whether an opioid is the most effective and appropriate treatment for a patient's pain, but also whether the risks of misuse, diversion, and other safety concerns can be managed effectively. Pain is a fact of life arising from many causes, not all of which respond favorably to opioids. In a subset of individuals, pain is an expression of underlying depression, anxiety, or addiction, and such conditions may actually worsen with opioids.[6-8]

Treating pain also is difficult because pain management has no single ideal outcome. Despite the prominence of pain intensity as a measure of efficacy in clinical trials and practice, everyday function and QOL are more important outcomes. Many patients value a treatment plan that offers realistic improvement in physical function, minimal side effects, and the possibility of regaining a sense of themselves. Most patients understand that 100% pain relief is not a realistic expectation. For chronic pain and well-established pain syndromes, pain intensity alone is an inadequate measure of the effectiveness of treatment.[9-14] Chronic pain is best viewed not as a vital sign but as a final common pathway, the end result of numerous biopsychosocial contributors that each must be addressed.[15]

# Total Pain

Pain is not an isolated sensory or emotional experience. Pain bidirectionally interacts with physical function, personality, mood, behavior, social relationships, and beliefs. Dame Cicely Saunders adopted the term *total pain* to describe the psychological, social, emotional, spiritual, and physical experience of pain; each domain contributes in a specific way to the individual pain experience. Some would like to broaden the concept to *total suffering,* which includes multiple symptoms. Beyond its physical dimension, pain threatens the *intactness* of a person.[16] Physical pain may be directly caused by illness, treatment, and comorbidities, but existential or spiritual pain arises from the impact on a person's sense of control, identity, justice, and meaning. Some people will have their faith threatened by pain while others will have their faith strengthened. Social pain results from loss of position and role within family and society. Pain and illness may put a patient in the difficult situation of having to shift from *doing* to *being.* Hard work and resilience are required to redefine one's sense of self to cope with psychosocial and spiritual challenges. Fear, depression, anxiety, and demoralization can intensify pain and make it more resistant to treatment. Suffering stemming from an existential sense of catastrophe, nihilism, or victimization won't respond to analgesics. Likewise, suffering associated with social isolation is opioid resistant.[17,18]

The diagnosis of a life-limiting illness opens the door to a heightened awareness of one's mortality, which may precipitate an experience of total pain.[19] Our death-denying modern society poorly equips us to handle the total pain of a life-limiting illness. Friends and family members may deny that a loved one is dying to protect themselves from loss and anticipatory grief. Death often is medicalized in acute care hospitals, where it is largely seen as only a physical experience. Patients may be encouraged to "fight on" and "not give up." Caregivers, friends, and family members may have an uncomfortable feeling of the salience of mortality when in the presence of loved ones with terminal illness and, as a result, treat them differently or simply avoid them altogether. As a carrot of hope when treatments are no longer beneficial, physicians may promise patients that they can resume potentially life-prolonging treatments when their condition improves. Patients may experience a cognitive dissonance between what they are told and the reality of their situation that increases psychological and social isolation. Despite advances in medical treatment, total pain can result in intense suffering.[20]

In coining the term *total pain,* Saunders applied the concept of patient centeredness to the understanding of pain and suffering, an approach that provides the foundation for holistic, interdisciplinary palliative care. Total pain is tied to a patient's personal narrative and ethnography, and all the suffering endured may be expressed simply as "pain." Saunders wrote, "Man by his very nature finds that he has to question the pain he endures and seek meaning in it."[21]

As early as 1959, Saunders recognized that pain could not be solely relieved by analgesics.[22] By 1967 the concept of total pain had evolved to the point that it influenced practice. Saunders wrote, "Pain demands the same analysis and consideration as an illness itself. It is the syndromes of pain rather than the syndromes of disease with which we are concerned."[23] In her work from 1968 through 1985, she recognized that chronic pain was particularly burdensome to patients. It posed a problem on the level of meaning—the persistence of chronic pain served no apparent purpose and could thus give rise to feelings of despair, isolation, and persecution. Acute pain made sense because it signaled an underlying problem and triggered a response that could protect function and survival, while chronic pain offered no such benefit.[24] She saw pain relief as the vital factor and the battleground on which to confront advocates for euthanasia. She demonstrated that modest dosages of potent opioids were helpful as one of several modalities to treat chronic cancer pain.

The end result of Saunders's approach was quite remarkable. Throughout the 1970s only 10% of patients admitted and treated at St. Christopher's Hospice needed more than 30 mg of diamorphine per day (equivalent to 30 mg of morphine daily). The degree of relief afforded by modest opioid dosages provided the opportunity to communicate and dialogue with patients on deeper issues, which led to further reductions in their pain.[25] Between the years 1972 and 1977 three-quarters of the 3,362 patients admitted to St. Christopher's Hospice had continuous uncontrolled pain prior to admission, but only 1% had poorly controlled pain thereafter.[26] However, to achieve these results, there was a cost for those providing the care; Saunders also recognized significant "staff pain" resulting from prolonged exposure to suffering patients and families. She wrote about what it takes for staff to stay engaged in treating total pain: "The resilience of those who continue to work in this field is won by a full understanding of what is happening and not by a retreat behind a technique."[26] Saunders left us with the wisdom that pain and suffering require assessment that is as thorough as the medical workup for its underlying illnesses.

# Chronic Pain

The Centers for Disease Control and Prevention (CDC) published guidelines in 2016 "to provide recommendations about opioid prescribing for primary care clinicians treating adult patients with chronic pain outside of active cancer treatment, palliative care, and end-of-life care."[27] However, one should not infer that opioids have greater efficacy or a better safety profile for patients with chronic pain who have cancer versus those without cancer.

As palliative care moves upstream in the course of cancer and other serious illnesses and is woven into the fabric of care from the point of diagnosis, palliative specialists will more frequently treat patients with chronic (longer than 3 months in duration) pain, including cancer survivors. This trend will call for a different approach than the eleventh-hour crisis intervention provided in hospices and acute care hospitals that characterized the early years of the hospice and palliative care movement.[28-30] Many people living with serious illness have chronic pain and are not immune to the long-term effects of opioids, including depression, hypogonadism, opioid-induced hyperalgesia, infections, falls, nonvertebral fractures, sleep-disordered breathing, cognitive dysfunction, sarcopenia, osteoporosis, and addiction.[31-39]

The opioid titration protocols recommended for patients with acute pain don't work as well when pain is chronic. The most effective treatments for chronic pain may not result in immediate substantial reductions in pain intensity.[13,40,41] The relief some patients experience simply because they *expect* a pain treatment to work is much greater with acute pain than it is with chronic pain. This enhanced placebo effect for patients with acute pain improves their response to opioid titration.[42] The literature is sparse about the general experience with long-term (longer than 12 months) opioid therapy for chronic noncancer pain, but what does exist is largely negative.[43] These trials demonstrate some reduction in pain intensity but have, for the most part, failed to show improved function or QOL. Pain outcomes between continuous and intermittent or low-dose opioids for chronic pain are similar relative to around-the-clock opioids, but those on around-the-clock opioids use three times more opioids per day and have greater psychological consternation with the use of opioids. Multiple studies have demonstrated greater risk for opioid-related death with high-dose daily opioids (100 mg morphine equivalents or more per day).[10,13,40,44] For patients on long-term opioids for noncancer pain, there is no relationship between opioid dose and pain scores.[11] Therefore, unlike for acute pain, those with chronic pain should not have pain intensity as the primary outcome measure but rather reduced pain interference, improved daily function, and reduced suffering.[10] Persistent helplessness and hopelessness may be a root cause of suffering for those with chronic pain, which gets communicated as "pain intensity."[10] The willingness to accept pain despite the perceptions of ongoing pain and engage in life activities (an internal locus of control) despite the presence of pain minimizes suffering by regaining a sense of self.[45-48]

## The "Average Patient" in Pain

It has long been recognized that there are large differences in outcomes among patients given the same analgesic therapy. In addition, many large, high-quality randomized controlled analgesic trials for chronic pain have produced negative findings despite encouraging results from preclinical and early clinical studies. One reason for negative human studies following promising animal studies is that patients entering clinical trials are much more heterogeneous than laboratory animals with respect to genetics, response to medications, and underlying mechanisms of pain.[49] This clinical heterogeneity obscures potential positive outcomes within certain subgroups of patients who suffer from the same pain syndrome. Within diagnostic categories, such as postherpetic neuralgia, there may be multiple underlying pain mechanisms and a host of patient-level variables that lead to marked interindividual variation in treatment responses.[49] This phenomenon is even more problematic in cancer pain. Most drugs attack one particular pain mechanism; however, pain is the sum result of multiple mechanisms and potential contributors—biological, sociological, and psychological. Precision medicine and personalized approaches to pain treatments will improve the clinical care of patients with persistent pain, and treatment based on pain phenotype will improve trial designs for potential analgesic drugs.[49] Current clinical trial designs, which involve patients with multiple pain phenotypes (as in cancer or neuropathic pain), are likely to miss potentially effective analgesic medications. A single estimate of effects in clinical trials, such as the change in mean pain intensity scores, is an average, group-level estimate. It cannot be presumed that every patient has an average improvement in pain and that an average response to treatment is the norm anticipated in practice. Individual patients vary greatly in the absolute benefit of analgesic therapy. Treatment has to be individualized. Some will benefit more than average while others will not benefit or may even be harmed. Current analgesic trial designs, which administer the same treatment to a wide range of patients and presume that all will resemble the patient behind the single-point average effect of treatment, do not reflect clinical reality. No one is an average patient; the wide range of treatment responses makes it impossible to predict how an individual patient will respond.[50]

# Pain Physiology

The International Association for the Study of Pain defines pain as "an unpleasant sensory and emotional experience associated with actual or potential tissue damage or described in terms of such damage."[51] Pain is defined as chronic if it lasts for 3 or more months after injury or beyond the time of normal tissue healing. Teleologically, pain either is protective, involving normal physiologic responses that prevent further injury, or it is an abnormal chronic pain state that has no protective purposes. This abnormal chronic pain state often is not explainable by pathology and is much more difficult to manage than acute pain.[52-54]

Pain classifications are divided most often into nociceptive (somatic or visceral) or neuropathic types or pain processing disorders such as fibromyalgia.[55-58] It is assumed that each has a distinct pathophysiology, yet evidence has shown that these different types of pain have common underlying mechanisms (see **Figure 1** and sidebar Mechanisms of Pain Transmission and Modulation below).

## The Science of Pain

### Mechanisms of Pain Transmission and Modulation

First-order A-delta and unmyelinated C-fibers synapse on the spinal cord, and second-order fibers cross over to the lateral spinothalamic tract and ascend to the reticular formation within the brainstem and to the thalamus and from there to various cortical centers (see Figure 1). These second-order sensory neurons connect to third-order neurons within limbic and cortical areas.[59] There is a "bottom-up" dampening of C-fiber neurotransmission within the superficial dorsal horn (lamina I-IV), which involves inhibitor interneurons within lamina II. This represents a "gate" that dampens nociceptive "traffic." There also is a "top-down" dampening of nociception through several brainstem nuclei.

One of the areas of "top-down" modulation is the subnucleus reticularis dorsalis (which is responsible for conditioned pain modulation). A second pathway is located within the periaqueductal grey (PAG) and rostral ventromedial medulla (RVM), which sends fibers down the spinal cord dorsolateral funiculus to produce postsynaptic inhibition on second-order neurons.[59-62] The PAG/RVM receives input from prefrontal cortex and rostral cingulate gyrus.

Loss of these "top-down" modulation functions are responsible for chronic pain as seen in fibromyalgia, in a subset of patients with neuropathic pain, chemotherapy neuropathy, and diabetic polyneuropathy.[62-71] "Top-down" inhibition can change to facilitation resulting in chronic pain from inflammation, neuropathic injury, and opioids (opioid-induced hyperalgesia).[62,72-76] The origins of "top-down" control through the PAG/RVM are from the prefrontal cortex and cingulate gyrus.

There is evidence that the anterior cingulate gyrus, which is responsible for metastatic bone pain hypersensitivity, has direct connections to the spinal cord. The involvement of prefrontal cortex and cingulate gyrus in pain processing also influences pain-related cognitive, motivational, and emotional responses. Opioids reduce pain by reducing the neurotransmission connectivity between affective and sensory parts of the brain such that patients have no impairment in locating pain, but the emotional trauma of pain is diminished.[77-79]

Classification systems for pain are based on etiology and pathogenesis. An effort to identify and characterize the etiology of the pain is one of the key elements to pain assessment (see Pain Assessment chapter on page 15). A number of classification systems based on etiology, pain pathophysiology, and temporal features (acute, chronic, or breakthrough) exist that identify distinct pain syndromes and guide treatment approaches. The pain initiator is a verifiable lesion or disorder that is likely to be perpetuating pain through ongoing direct tissue injury or inflammation. When the etiology is identified, analgesic and disease-modifying therapies are started as part of a comprehensive and coordinated plan. Disease-modifying therapy may consist of radiation to a bony metastasis, surgery, or systemic antitumor therapy.

The underlying mechanisms of pain are increasingly being understood as complex neuronal dynamic phenomena in which the resulting neuroplastic changes sustain pain even after the inciting injury is no longer present and tissues have healed.[18] Two broad, oversimplified categories of pain—nociceptive (which includes both somatic and visceral pain, despite differences in neurosensory processing) and neuropathic—conventionally are accepted as a classification and are found to be useful in directing treatment choices. Although basic science research in bone pain[80] and neuropathic injury[81] suggest that such labels are an oversimplification of multiple complex mechanisms, this classification, and the identification of cancer pain syndromes, are useful in practice.[82]

Bone pain from cancer has been assumed to have a distinctly different pain mechanism than neuropathic pain, yet bone metastases will generate neuropathic pain as measured by the Self-Reported Leeds Assessment of Neuropathic Symptoms and Signs Scale.[83] Patients with neuropathic pain from bone metastases will have more severe pain intensity as measured by the Brief Pain Inventory, and their pain will be less responsive to analgesics.[83] Acute inflammation causes pain hypersensitivity by inactivating the pain-dampening function of the ventrolateral prefrontal cortex, rostral cingulate cortex, and PAG/RVM. This pathway also is commonly altered in the same manner with neuropathic pain.[84] Peripheral inflammation, bone metastases, and neuropathic pain all produce a neuroinflammatory response with activated glia.[85-89]

# Figure 1. The Anatomy of Pain

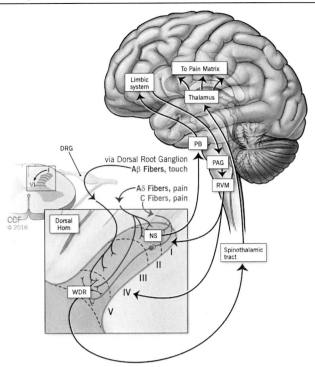

*Nociceptors in peripheral tissues represent the distal part of first-order afferent neurons. First-order affer-ent neurons consist of small-diameter fibers, either unmyelinated (C-fibers) or sparsely myelinated A-delta fibers. A-delta fibers promote quick sensations of acute pain triggering withdrawal while C-fibers propa-gate in a slow way. C-fibers can have prolonged action-potentials, which summate afferent input over time and induce dull pain.*

*First-order sensory neurons merge into Lissauer Tract and enter the dorsal horn to synapse with sec-ond-order neurons and wide dynamic range neurons. After direct or indirect interactions with projection neurons within the dorsal horn of the spinal cord , second-order neurons become part of the spinothalamic tract which projects to thalamus, parabrachial nucleus as well as to the periaqueductal gray (PAG), limbic system, and hypothalamus. The parabrachial nucleus projects to multiple other structures within the limbic system. The thalamus receives projections from the spinothalamic tract. Lateral thalamic projections go to sensory cortex for pain discrimination and the medial projections to the anterior cingulate gyrus and insular cortex, which is involved with the affective and motivational components to pain.*

*Descending pain modulation comes from a number of supraspinal sites, including the periaqueductal grey (PAG) and rostral ventromedial medulla (RVM). The PAG-RVM through the dorsal funiculus preferentially suppresses nociceptive input from spinal C-fibers. Cells governing bidirectional control of pain within the PAG/RVM (on-cells for facilitation, off-cells for inhibition) are recruited by higher structures important in fear, illness, and psychological stress*

*Reprinted with permission, Cleveland Clinic Center for Medical Art & Photography. © 2016. All Rights Reserved.*

Nociceptive pain may be somatic or visceral.[90] Inflammatory pain is sometimes distinguished on the basis of identifiable inflammation (eg, heat, redness, elevated Westergren sedimentation rate, elevated C-reactive protein, low serum albumin, high neutrophil to lymphocyte ratio) and presumably indirectly activates nociceptors (such as through prostaglandins).

Because of shared mechanisms of pain, such classifications of pain may be inadequate to guide analgesic therapies. As we begin to understand the mechanisms of pain, we start to realize the overlapping nature of pain classifications. This also means that analgesic choices may more reasonably be chosen based on the particular pain phenotype than by disease. For example, gabapentin is used for neuropathic pain but also can be useful to treat bone pain from cancer.[91-93] In animal models, increased temporal summation and wind-up by quantitative testing can be targeted successfully with gabapentinoids and conditions of impaired pain modulation by duloxetine.[61,67,94]

Pain phenotypes are determined by uncovering dysfunctional nociceptive processing through quantitative sensory testing. This may be a better way of selecting analgesics than choices based on disease or nociceptive- versus neuropathic-based classifications.

## Cancer-Related Bone Pain

Cancer-related bone pain is the end result of a complex array of mechanisms. Cancers shift the balance of bone-matrix turnover toward osteolysis through activation of osteoclasts. Net resorption of bone disrupts the bone microarchitecture, reducing bone strength, increasing the risk for fracture, and placing individuals at risk for hypercalcemia.[95,96] Cancer-associated osteoclast activation occurs by way of upregulation of receptor activator of nuclear factor kappa-B-receptor and its ligand (RANK-RANKL). RANKL is released by tumors, tumor associated T-cells, and osteoblasts.[97] Tumor cells also produce parathyroid hormone–related protein, which increases the release of RANKL. Osteolysis reduces local pH. Acidosis stimulates acid-sensing ion channels (ASIC) and vanilloid receptors, which activate sensory afferents within the bone and periosteum, causing pain and hypersensitivity around the bone involved with cancer. Bisphosphonates inhibit osteoclasts, and denosumab (a monoclonal antibody) blocks RANK-RANKL binding, resulting in reduced cancer-related bone destruction and pain.[98,99]

Cancer within the bone marrow and periosteum destroys sensory fibers, causing a neuropathic pain and a neuroplastic response that results in reorganization, sprouting of nerve endings, and neuroma formation.[100-102] This reorganization contributes to spontaneous and breakthrough pain episodes. Sensory afferent reorganization is caused by increased release of nerve-growth factor.[103,104]

Nerve growth factor not only increases sprouting but also increases expression of substance P, calcitonin gene–related peptide, sodium channels, and ASIC within dorsal root ganglion, resulting in a central sensitization.[105,106] Tanezumab, a monoclonal antibody against nerve growth factor reported in 2014, shows promise, experimentally, at reducing cancer-related bone pain.[95,107]

Spinal cord changes due to cancer-related bone pain include expression of dynorphin (an endogenous kappa opiate), neuroinflammation with activation of microglia and astrocytes, increased expression of N-Methyl-D-asparate (NMDA) subunits, and activation of NMDA receptors. Phenotypic changes occur in neuron populations, resulting in increased wide dynamic range neurons deeper in the dorsal laminae and subsequent increased temporal summation.[89] Wide dynamic range neurons travel through the parabrachial nucleus rather than synapse on the sensory cortex; they synapse within the limbic system, which generates emotional/affective responses to pain.

Cancer bone pain is relatively resistant to opioid analgesics, which may be related to the development of neuroinflammation. Neuroinflammation reduces opioid analgesia.[108,109] In addition, mu opioid receptors are epigenetically down-modulated in the dorsal root ganglia of the innervating dermatome of the cancerous bone.

## Neuropathic Pain

Neuropathic pain is caused by an injury, lesion, or disease to the somatosensory system (**Table 1**).[110] Clinically, neuropathic pain occurs in an area of sensory deficit.[55] Approximately 40% of individuals with cancer are affected by neuropathic pain. People with neuropathic pain have poorer cognition and physical and social functioning than individuals without neuropathic pain.[111] There are four specific criteria to the clinical description:

1. pain in a distinct neuroanatomical distribution
2. a history of trauma, surgery, or tumor affecting the somatosensory system
3. confirmatory tests demonstrating negative (eg, sensory and motor deficits) and positive (eg, hypersensitivity) sensory signs within the innervated territory
4. diagnostic tests that confirm a lesion or disease entity underlying the neuropathic pain.[112]

Positive symptoms of neuropathy include paresthesia and/or dysesthesia, allodynia (pain triggered by non-noxious stimuli), hyperalgesia (exaggerated responsive to a painful stimulus), and spontaneous pain. Allodynia can be dynamic if triggered by brushing or static if evoked by pressure or punctate (needle) stimuli.[56]

The words people use to describe their pain differ more with the experience of neuropathic pain than they do with nociceptive pain. These "core" neuropathic pain descriptors include terms such as burning, electric-shock-like, tingling, and increased sensitivity, among others.[129] Other aberrant sensations that may accompany the pain and disturbances of sensation, such as allodynia (pain from light touch or mild pressure) or hyperalgesia (increased response to a noxious stimulus),[130] may be prominent. Questionnaires particular for neuropathic pain (Neuropathic Pain Scale, Neuropathic Pain Symptom Inventory) are built on sensory descriptors.[131] These questionnaires have demonstrated that neuropathic pain based on disease is actually a heterogeneous collection of different pain mechanisms that may include as many as five

## Table 1. Mechanisms Contributing to Neuropathic Pain

Ectopy from injured nerve and upregulation of sodium channels[113,114]

Upregulation of receptors in surrounding uninjured C-fibers, resulting in increased heat-sensing channels and subsequently heat hypersensitivity and burning pain[115]

Phenotype switches of nociceptors to wide dynamic range neurons within spinal cord[116,117]

Increased production/upregulation of substance P, calcitonin gene-related peptide, and brain-derived neurotrophic factor in large-sized neurons resulting in increased excitatory neurotransmission[118,119]

Loss of potassium channels and impaired repolarization of neurons[120,121]

Reduced expression of opioid receptors[122]

Collateral sprouting of peripheral afferents into sympathetic fibers within the dorsal root ganglion and primary afferents within the spinal cord resulting in sympathetic mediated pain[123-125]

Loss of GABAergic inhibitory interneurons within the spinal cord superficial dorsal lamina[126]

Changes within the PAG/RVM causing facilitation rather than inhibition of pain[127]

Neuroinflammation and activation of microglia and astrocytes resulting in upregulation of interleukins and chemokines and thus reduced glutamate transporters, increased neurotransmission via NMDA receptors, and increased prostaglandin production[128]

---

different components or dimensions.[132] Conditions such as cancer, neuropathic pain, diabetic neuropathy, and postherpetic neuralgia may display multiple pain phenotypes with different underlying mechanisms of pain despite being classified under a single entity. Specific combinations of symptoms and signs reflect different underlying pathophysiological mechanisms. The empiric use of analgesics for neuropathic pain often leads to therapeutic failure; neuropathic pain is less responsive to opioid therapy.[133]

Examples of chronic neuropathic pain syndromes include postherpetic neuralgia, postsurgical painful mononeuropathies (eg, postmastectomy and postthoracotomy pain syndromes), chemotherapy-induced painful polyneuropathy, malignant plexopathy, and phantom pain syndromes. Cancers also can produce paraneoplastic sensory neuropathies or mixed motor and sensory neuropathies.

The recognition of a cancer pain syndrome by history and physical examination guides additional assessment, including radiographic imaging and treatment, and clarifies prognosis if new in onset. If recognized early, one may be able to prevent complications or offer reassurance to patients who have interpreted their comorbid noncancer pain as cancer progression. Numerous nociceptive and neuropathic pain syndromes associated with cancer have been described in observational studies.[134]

There are multiple mechanisms of neuropathic cancer pain (see Table 1). Neuropathic pain can be due to nerve compression, deafferentation nerve damage, and sympathetically induced pain. Tumors can infiltrate nerves, cause perineural inflammation, or disrupt neuron integrity and transmission via ischemia. Deafferentation pain occurs with prolonged tumor infiltration. Sympathetically maintained pain is associated with abnormal sweating, trophic skin changes, and allodynia, which is usually not in a dermatomal distribution.[135,136]

Surgery, chemotherapy, and radiation may induce neuropathic injury and pain, which can persist through survivorship. Commonly used chemotherapy drugs such as oxaliplatin, carboplatin, cisplatin, paclitaxel, docetaxel, bortezomib, lenalidomide, thalidomide, and vinca alkaloids will produce neuropathic pain.[137] Oxaliplatin and paclitaxel can cause acute neuropathic pain.

It is unlikely that a single analgesic will block the multitude of mechanisms that result in neuropathic pain; combinations of analgesics are likely needed to be able to effectively treat it.[138-140]

## Somatic Pain

Somatic pain is caused by injury to the skin, other soft tissues, bones, or joints. Deep somatic pain typically is localized and described as aching, stabbing, throbbing, or "squeezing." Superficial somatic pain is usually sharper and may have a burning or pricking sensation. Examples of somatic pain include arthritis, cutaneous wounds, and tumor invasion of soft tissues.

Metastatic bone disease typically is labeled as somatic nociceptive pain, notwithstanding some data demonstrating a fundamental neuropathic process involved in at least some types.[80] Bone pain intensifies with movement (especially weight bearing), is often tender to palpation, and is often described as deep and aching. Bone pain requires a particularly careful assessment.[141] If there is severe pain during any weight-bearing activity, a radiograph may reveal an actual or potential pathologic fracture for which orthopedic stabilization or radiation therapy may be needed.

## Visceral Pain

Visceral pain presumably results from activation of nociceptors in the viscera by compression, obstruction, infiltration, ischemia, stretching, or inflammation. When injury involves a hollow viscus, the pain usually is not well-localized and often is described as cramping, gnawing, squeezing, or pressure. Depending on the structures involved, the pain may improve or worsen with eating or bowel movements or distension of the bladder or bowel. Injury to some visceral tissues, such as organ capsules, mesentery or other fascia, or the heart or pancreas, produces pain that usually is described as sharp or stabbing, referring to well-described patterns of certain anatomic areas.

## Nocebo and Placebo Responses

One complicating factor in analgesic trials is the *placebo response,* a reduction in pain caused by the patient's belief that the medication will work. Similarly, a patient who fears a treatment or distrusts the medical team may experience a *nocebo response,* an adverse event triggered by the negative expectation.[142-147] Placebo ("I shall please") powerfully influences the brain in different pathological conditions (eg, pain, anxiety, depression, motor disorders) and in different immune and endocrine systems.[148-150] Placebo pain responses are blocked by naloxone; responses appear to be mediated through the PAG/RVM.[151-154] A main assumption is that placebo analgesia is caused by the actions of endogenous opioids. Alternatively, placebo analgesia may be related to an altered constitutional activity of opioid receptors independent of endogenous opioid ligands.[155-157] Placebo responses double analgesic responses and are equivalent to as much as 8 mg of parenteral morphine. Expectation of benefits is key to placebo responses.[158] Expectation activates the endogenous opioid system and pain-modulating networks and reduces pain transmission in specific brain regions that can be visualized by functional magnetic resonance imaging (fMRI).[159] Subtle subconscious events of which patients are unaware can elicit placebo responses.[160,161] Placebo responses can occur with other symptoms. In one postoperative study, placebo responses accounted for the entire diazepam benefit when treating anxiety.[162]

Nocebo ("I shall harm") effects are generated when treatment is delivered within a negative psychosocial context. It also has biologic correlates.[163] Examples include worsening symptoms after a negative diagnosis, bad news about disease relapse, or a negative expectation about the disease course. Nocebo responses occur when patients distrust medical personnel or procedures. Unwanted side effects and adverse effects occur because of negative expectations.[164,165] Negative health warnings by mass media have a perceived impact on symptoms of many individuals.[166] Biologically, cholecystokinin is an important mediator of the nocebo response that is blocked by cholecystokinin-B receptor antagonists.[144,167,168] Nocebo responses are not influenced by naloxone. Cholecystokinin is not involved in the anxiety component of the nocebo effect. Benzodiazepines reduce anticipatory anxiety responses to pain. Cholecystokinin receptor blockers are not analgesics in the usual sense, but blockers reduce nocebo-induced pain.[163]

# Pain Assessment

## Clinical Situation

### Maggie

Maggie is a 65-year-old woman with a history of metastatic breast cancer. She had a right total mastectomy with lymph node dissection and now has a single metastasis to her fourth lumbar vertebrae. She is undergoing cisplatin-based chemotherapy and radiation and is referred to a palliative care clinic for help with pain management. Maggie is tearful as she shares the multiple pains she is experiencing, which include constant dull aching pain in her lower back, chest wall pain at the site of her mastectomy, and sharp shooting pain down her right arm. The numbness and tingling in both hands and feet started soon after the chemotherapy. The right arm lymphedema and pain are new. She tearfully reports that her pain has worsened her mood, sleep, and appetite. Maggie is fearful that her cancer is returning because of her worsening pain. The resident who is rotating with you asks, "Where do we start with this patient?"

 When approaching a patient with multiple sources of pain, the following questions may be helpful:

- How long have you had your pain?
- Can you describe your pain? What is the quality of your pain?
- Does your pain have a continuous or episodic character?
- How badly has your pain adversely influenced your everyday life?
- Has there been anything you have found that has relieved your pain?
- What do you think is causing your pain or pains?
- What are your greatest fears?
- Are you able to tell me which pain is causing you the most trouble, such as interfering with activity, sleep, personal care, interest in doing things you normally need to do, want to do, like to do?

Maggie shares with you that her husband left her after learning of her cancer, and she is experiencing a great deal of demoralization and loneliness as a result. Though she is lonely and needs social support, her children live out of state, and she doesn't want to "bother" her friends. She becomes tearful in the office and says, "I just don't understand why this is happening to me. What did I do to deserve this cancer?"

What elements from Maggie's history point to the following types of pain?

- Emotional
- Social
- Spiritual
- Existential

How do you explore Maggie's total pain?

How difficult is it to do this if Maggie's physical pain is either untreated or undertreated?

## Objectives

Patients with serious illness experiencing significant pain should receive a systematic and comprehensive assessment that captures the multiple dimensions of pain.[169] The assessment should be comprehensive enough to develop a plan of care for pain management, including domains of "total pain" such as psychosocial and spiritual concerns that contribute to suffering and the burden of illness (**Table 2**). Depending on the history and physical examination, laboratory testing or diagnostic imaging may be indicated to determine the sources of physical pain and identify treatment options.

## Components of Multidimensional Pain Assessment

Taking a thorough history requires empathetic listening and the exploration of sufficient information from the patient to fully characterize each pain complaint. Patients frequently have multiple pains. Standardized pain assessment tools such as the Brief Pain Inventory or similar questionnaires systematically record the pain characteristics and their impact on cognitive function, mood, sleep, appetite, physical activities, social functioning, and overall QOL. When not using a standard questionnaire, some clinicians find the mnemonic PQRST to be a helpful prompt (**Table 3**). A numerical, categorical, or visual analog scale may be used to track changes in pain severity over time and in response to treatment. It also is important to regularly reassess the impact of pain on function, sleep, mood, and anxiety. If opioid therapy is being considered, patients should be asked about any personal history of drug, alcohol, or tobacco abuse; family history of drug abuse; or history of being abused as a child. Patients receiving pharmacological therapies systematically should be asked about side effects.

### Assessing Pain Severity

Pain severity (the "S" in the PQRST mnemonic) is the dominant factor that determines the effects of pain on patients and the urgency of treatment. Because pain is subjective and lacks

## Table 2. Key Objectives of a Pain Assessment[170]

1. To characterize the multiple dimensions of the pain (eg, using the PQRST mnemonic—see Table 3)
2. To formulate an understanding of the nature of the pain
   » Etiology
   » Inferred pathophysiology
   » Pain syndrome
3. To characterize the impact of the pain on quality-of-life domains
   » Effect on physical functioning and well-being
   » Effect on mood, coping, and related aspects of psychological well-being
   » Effect on role functioning and social and familial relationships
   » Effect on sleep, mood, vitality, and sexual function
4. To clarify the extent of the underlying disease, planned treatment, and prognosis
5. To clarify the nature and quality of prior testing and past treatments
6. To elucidate medical comorbidities
7. To elucidate psychiatric comorbidities
   » Substance use history
   » Depression and anxiety disorders
   » Personality disorders
8. To determine other needs for palliative care interventions
   » Other symptoms
   » Distress related to psychosocial or spiritual concerns
   » Caregiver burden and concrete needs
   » Problems in communication, care coordination, and goal setting

*Reprinted from* The Lancet, *377(9784), by RK Portenoy, Treatment of Cancer Pain, 2236-2247, Copyright ©2011, with permission from Elsevier.*

## Table 3. PQRST Pain Assessment Mnemonic[171]

| | |
|---|---|
| **P** | Palliative, provocative factors: What makes the pain better or worse? |
| **Q** | Quality (word descriptors such as "burning" or "stabbing") |
| **R** | Region, radiation, referral (radicular, nonradicular pattern): Where does it hurt? Does the pain move or travel? |
| **S** | Severity (pain intensity rating scales or word descriptors) |
| **T** | Temporal factors (onset, duration, daily fluctuations): When did it start? Is it constant and/or intermittent? How long does it last? Is it better or worse at certain times of the day? |

*From Nonmalignant pain in palliative medicine (p. 934), by S Weinstein, in D Walsh, R Fainsinger, K Foley, et al. (eds.),* Palliative Medicine, *2009, Philadelphia: Saunders. © 2009 by Elsevier. Reprinted with permission.*

objective biological markers, the gold standard in assessment is the patient's self-report. Validated scales that assess pain severity are either unidimensional or multidimensional.

Examples of unidimensional pain scales (**Figure 2**) include a simple verbal rating scale (eg, mild, moderate, severe) or a numeric rating scale (NRS).[172] The NRS (eg, "on a scale from 0 to 10, where 0 equals no pain and 10 equals the worst possible pain, how severe is your pain right now?") may be administered verbally or in writing. Other scales such as the Visual Analog Scale (VAS) or a pictorial scale (eg, the Wong-Baker FACES™ Pain Rating Scale, developed specifically for children [**Figure 3**],[173] or the Iowa Pain Thermometer [**Figure 4**][174,175]) are administered using a written tool. Patients from different cultures may find it easier to respond to individualized symbols for pain, such as a series of pictures of fires that become increasingly larger. Older adults may prefer using pain terminology such as *discomfort, aching, hurting,* or *soreness.* Regardless of the scale used, it is important to use the same scale and terminology with the patient consistently to ensure reliability.

The key requirements of pain measurement include the following:

1. Use the patient's preferred pain terminology and the same pain scale each time.
2. If possible, have the same clinician assess pain each time.
3. When assessing pain intensity, also provide the time frame (eg, "pain right now," "pain during the past day"), and consider asking about more than one descriptor (eg, "pain on average during the past day," "pain at its worst during the past day"). It is more reliable to use the time frame "over the past 24 hours" than the time frame "now." Alternatively, use the "worst" pain, the "least" pain, and the "average" pain over the last 24 hours.

Multidimensional pain scales such as the McGill Pain Questionnaire (MPQ) and the Brief Pain Inventory (BPI) assess pain severity and other pain characteristics.[176] The MPQ evaluates pain qualities, and the BPI focuses on pain's influence on mood and function. These instruments are sometimes used in clinical practice in their entirety and they are consistently used in research.[176] The longer it takes patients to complete the tool, the less likely it is to be completed. The tool should be written at the appropriate education level so that patients can understand the questions. People who are not familiar with healthcare terminology and those who are fatigued, frail, or have mild cognitive deficits or dementia may not understand the tool.

Some multidimensional scales, such as the Edmonton Symptom Assessment Scale (ESAS), assess the presence and severity of a combination of physical and psychological symptoms, providing a snapshot of the total symptom burden experience.[177] Summing the severity scores of the ESAS yields an overall symptom burden score. Some scales are copyrighted and cannot be used without permission. The ESAS is available to use without a need to ask for copyright permission, is validated and reliable, and has the ability to measure clinically meaningful changes in symptom severity over time.

# Figure 2. Unidimensional Pain Scales Compared with the Faces Pain Scale-Revised

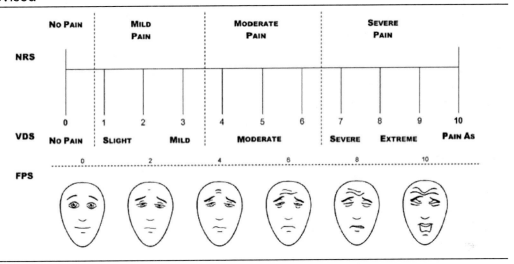

FPS, Faces Pain Scale; NRS, numeric rating scale; VDS, verbal descriptor scale.

FPS instructions: When giving the following instructions, say "hurt" or "pain," whichever seems right for a particular child. "These faces show how much something can hurt. This face (point to left-most face) shows no pain. The faces show more and more pain (point to each from left to right) up to this one (point to right-most face)—it shows very much pain. Point to the face that shows how much you hurt (right now)." Score the chosen face 0, 2, 4, 6, 8, or 10, counting left to right so 0 = no pain and 10 = very much pain. Do not use words such as "happy" and "sad." This scale is intended to measure how children feel inside, not how their face looks.

From The Faces Pain Scale–Revised: toward a common metric in pediatric pain measurement, by CL Hicks, CL von Baeyer, P Spafford, I van Korlaar, and B Goodenough, 2001, Pain, 93, 173-183. The Faces Pain Scale for the self-assessment of the severity of pain experienced by children: development, initial validation and preliminary investigation for ratio scale properties, by D Bieri, R Reeve, GD Champion, L Addicoat, and J Ziegler, 1990, Pain, 41, 139-150. © 2001 by the International Association for the Study of Pain. Reprinted with permission.

# Figure 3. Wong-Baker FACES™ Pain Rating Scale

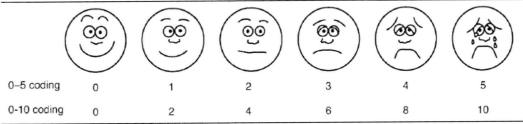

From Wong's Essentials of Pediatric Nursing, 7th ed. (p. 1259), by MJ Hockenberry, D Wilson, and ML Winkelstein, 2005, 1259. St. Louis: Mosby. © 2005 by Mosby. Reprinted with permission.

# Figure 4. Iowa Pain Thermometer

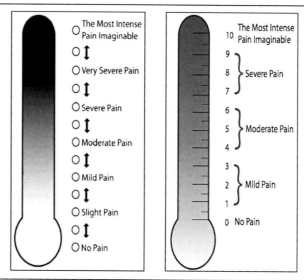

## Assessing Pain Location

Pain may be well- or poorly localized or have more than one location with different characteristics. The location of pain is assessed by asking the patient to pinpoint precisely where on his or her body the pain is located or, alternatively, on a body diagram (such as that found on the BPI). This should include areas where the pain radiates.

## Assessing Pain Quality

Pain quality (the "Q" in the PQRST mnemonic) is characterized by descriptors such as sharp, deep, crampy, tingling, and burning that can help differentiate somatic, visceral, and neuropathic pain mechanisms. Somatic nociceptive pain is usually described as sharp or dull, well-localized, aching, or as a squeezing sensation. Visceral pain is usually poorly localized, described as a deep pressure–like sensation, and may be associated with cramps. Neuropathic pain is described as burning, tingling, electrical, stabbing, or "pins and needles." It is usually associated with areas of neurologic deficits (numbness, motor weakness.) Pain is not infrequently a complex mixture of nociceptive and neuropathic types. Patients may not know how to describe the quality of pain they are experiencing, so clinicians may facilitate assessment by providing the patient a list of potential descriptors to help characterize the pain quality. Funicular pain (ie, pain that is funnel-like and squeezing, such as on an upper or lower extremity) is a sign of an impending spinal cord compression. Muscle cramps experienced by individuals with cancer more often are neuropathic in nature rather than myopathic.

## Assessing Temporal Features of Pain

The "T" in the PQRST mnemonic refers to temporal aspects of the pain experience. Most patients with advanced illness have some degree of constant or background pain punctuated with episodes of greater severity known as breakthrough pain. Patients with cancer frequently report a worsening of their pain at night. Effective assessment and treatment requires attention to both continuous (background) and breakthrough pain. Some patients only have episodic pain, either precipitated by activity (incident pain) or occurring spontaneously, such as abdominal cramping or "lightning-like" neuropathic discharges. When asking about breakthrough pain, details related to frequency, onset, duration, predictability, and impact are essential for determining the best treatment strategy. Breakthrough pain can be spontaneous or incident to activity, and it should not be confused with end-of-dose-failure pain, which occurs close to the time the next dose of an around-the-clock analgesic is due and reflects inadequate dosing to keep the continuous background pain under control.

## Assessing Palliative Factors

Patients often try to ease their pain by changing position, using heat or cold, or taking over-the-counter medications. Certain positions, activities, or events may affect the severity pain and provide clues to its underlying mechanism. For example, patients with cancer, pain that gets worse when they cough or perform a Valsalva maneuver may be due to metastases to the spine or ribs, while pain worsened by taking a deep breath would point instead to involvement of the diaphragm, pleura, or liver. On the other hand, patients with pancreatic cancer and retroperitoneal metastases may find that they can lessen their pain by bending forward in a fetal position.

## History Assessment

As part of the clinical history, information about prior episodes of pain and its treatment and the current impact of pain on various domains of function should be elucidated. Assessment for the presence of patient- and family-related barriers to pain management—such as fear of opioid addiction and adverse effects, the belief that increased pain means disease progression, and the presence of depression—is important because those barriers may lead to underreporting of pain and therapeutic nonadherence.[178,179]

A psychosocial assessment should be performed, both to assess the meaning of pain for the patient and family and to determine if other issues deserve attention in the broader plan of palliative care. A patient's previous experience, culture, social milieu, personality, and situational stressors may influence how pain is expressed. Exploring pain and other stressors with patients may reveal clues about their usual coping strategies and resilience, which should inform their plan of care.

Given the reliance on opioid therapy as a key approach to the treatment of pain in medically ill patients, it is extremely important to ask about the patient's previous and current relationships with potentially abusable drugs, including alcohol, controlled prescription medications, and illicit drugs. When the family history is queried, it is equally important to determine whether drug abuse has occurred in the immediate family.[180,181] The use of medications such as opioids in a manner outside their prescribed purpose as a way to manage the stress associated with a terminal diagnosis such as cancer has been called "chemical coping." Any patient with a past history of alcohol or drug abuse is more likely than others to have a maladaptive coping strategy involving opioids when faced with the stressors of serious illness. Studies suggest an association between chemical coping and high pain expression, opioid dose escalation, and the inability to discontinue opioids after resolution of the painful condition.[182-185] Although the exact frequency of chemical coping in the palliative care population is not known, one retrospective study found 18% of patients with advanced cancer seen by a palliative care service were diagnosed with chemical coping but only 4% of cases were documented in the medical records.[186] For early identification of patients at risk for chemical coping, there are several brief validated screening tools that can be used as part of the initial evaluation of patients with pain.[187-189]

### Patient Expectations and Goals

Clinicians must ascertain the patient's and family's knowledge of expectations and goals for pain management when determining appropriate therapy. Patients with life-threatening illnesses frequently harbor anxieties and fears and may be reluctant to discuss them for a host of reasons. To position pain management within the broader scope of palliative care, clinicians should ask and listen for clues about the presence of psychological, social, and spiritual distress that may be contributing to suffering and amplifying the pain experience. By providing a nonjudgmental and compassionate presence, physicians and other members of the care team can provide a therapeutic environment that builds trust and relieves suffering, which may do more good than any further medical tests or treatments could.

### Patient Concerns

When assessing the complex contributors to the suffering and illness burden experienced by patients and their families, it is useful to include open-ended questions during history taking. However, patients with severe physical pain may have limited ability to engage, and in such cases lengthier discussion should be pursued only after achieving a higher level of comfort. Examples of questions that may either illuminate the pain report or elicit concerns other than pain include the following:

- When people become seriously ill, they usually find themselves wondering why it happened to them. When you think about this, what comes to mind?
- When you think about the next few weeks or months, what are some concerns that first come to mind? What things concern you more than others?
- When you think back over the years, what are some of your happiest times? Saddest times?

- What has given you strength in the past? What gives you strength now? What do you wish could happen to give you more strength?
- How has this illness affected you emotionally? What has been particularly difficult? Has anything been more (or less) difficult than you thought it might be?
- How is your family coping with this illness? Can you tell me something about what is going on with them? What are some of your concerns about your family?

The information acquired through this detailed history taking is necessary to establish working hypotheses about the nature of the pain and contextual information essential to optimize the plan of care. The next step, an examination, provides additional information about the pain itself and an assessment of the disease status, comorbidities, and general physical condition of the patient.[190]

### Assessing Pain in Patients with Cognitive Impairment

When patients are unable to communicate, behavioral observations and proxy reports from caregivers substitute for self-report of pain intensity. Behavioral cues suggestive of pain or distress include verbal cues (eg, crying, moaning, and groaning) as well as nonverbal cues such as facial expressions (eg, grimacing, biting lips), body movements, clenching of fists, restlessness, guarding, and social interactions (eg, being withdrawn, wanting to spend time in bed). Many staff-administered behavioral instruments have been validated for use with patients with severe cognitive impairment. When considering proxy reports from family members or caregivers, it is important to keep in mind that these have not always been shown to be in concordance with the patient's report.[191-193] Thus, clinicians should use proxy reports in combination with behavioral cues when assessing pain for patients with severe cognitive impairments. When in doubt, a trial of analgesics may be warranted.

### Assessing Pain in the Intensive Care Unit

Assessing pain in the intensive care unit (ICU) is a challenge. Two pain behavior instruments have been tested for reliability, validity, and feasibility for use in ICUs: the Pain Behavior Scale and the Critical-Care Pain Observation Tool.[194] Other tools include the Pain Assessment, Intervention, and Notation (PAIN) algorithm and a Pain Behaviors Checklist.[195] According to Puntillo and colleagues, when established tools are insufficient, alternative methods to augment a pain evaluation should be considered. These methods include completing a pain risk profile using surrogates or performing an analgesic trial.[196] When working with deeply sedated patients in the ICU, neither verbal nor behavioral measures are feasible. In these cases, physiologic changes such as tachycardia and hypertension are used to track the potential effects of noxious stimuli.

## Physical Examination

In many cases a physical examination (**Table** 4) begins with vital signs. However, the physiological signs associated with acute pain such as elevated blood pressure, respiratory rate, and pulse typically disappear when pain is prolonged and thus are unreliable indicators when pain becomes chronic. It is common for patients experiencing severe chronic pain to have entirely normal vital signs and, moreover, to not look like they are in pain.

In most cases, the examination should include both a neurological and musculoskeletal assessment. Pain associated with neurological findings may suggest neuropathic mechanisms; the absence of neurological findings, however, does not exclude this diagnosis. Pain that is reproduced by mechanical factors such as joint motion, weight bearing, or gait suggests an etiology involving the musculoskeletal system. In the soft tissues, one may palpate muscle spasms or discrete trigger points, which, when stimulated, refer pain to another site.

### Table 4. Physical Examination[171]

General Inspection
- Patient's appearance and vital signs
- Evidence of abnormalities such as weight loss, muscle atrophy, deformities, trophic changes

Pain Site Assessment
- Inspect the pain sites for abnormal appearance or color of overlying skin, change of contour, or visible muscle spasm.
- Palpate the sites for tenderness and texture.
- Use percussion to elicit, reproduce, or evaluate the pain and any tenderness on palpation.
- Determine the effects of physical factors such as position, pressure, and motion.

Neurological Examination
- Mental status: level of alertness, higher cognitive functions, affect
- Cranial nerves
- Sensory system: light touch and pinprick test to assess for allodynia, evoked dysesthesia, hypoesthesia/hyperesthesia, hypoalgesia/hyperalgesia, hyperpathia
- Motor system: muscle bulk and tone, abnormal movements, manual motor testing, reflexes
- Coordination, station, and gait

Musculoskeletal Examination
- Body type, posture, and overall symmetry
- Abnormal spine curvature, limb alignment, and other deformities
- Range of motion (spine, extremities)
- For muscles in the neck, upper extremities, trunk, and lower extremities: Observe for any abnormalities such as atrophy, hypertrophy, irritability, tenderness, and trigger points.

*From Nonmalignant pain in palliative medicine (p. 934), by S Weinstein, in D Walsh, R Fainsinger, K Foley, et al. (Eds.), Palliative Medicine, 2009, Philadelphia: Saunders. © 2009 by Elsevier. Reprinted with permission.*

# Review of Data

The pain evaluation concludes with a review of available laboratory and imaging studies (**Table 5**). When caring for imminently dying patients, further information of this type is not actionable and should be eschewed. At other times, however, the nature of the pain and goals of care indicate the need for additional tests to diagnosis the cause of the pain, evaluate the extent of disease, and determine the feasibility of disease-modifying therapy or special pain management procedures (see Table 5). If a patient has a long history of chronic pain, a critical evaluation of the history, findings on examination, and imaging studies may be necessary to determine whether the etiology of a pain problem is related to a preexisting or comorbid condition rather than the life-threatening illness.[197]

## Table 5. Diagnostic Testing for Pain[171]

| Types of Tests | Uses |
|---|---|
| Screening laboratory tests: CBC, chemistry profile (eg, electrolytes, liver, enzymes, BUN, creatinine), urinalysis, ESR | Screen for medical illnesses, organ dysfunction |
| Disease-specific laboratory tests (includes autoantibodies, sickle cell test) | Autoimmune disorders, SCD |
| Imaging studies: radiographs, CT, MRI, US, myelography | Detection of tumors, other structural abnormalities |
| Diagnostic procedures: lumbar puncture for CSF analysis | Detection of various CNS illnesses |
| Electrophysiological tests: EMG (direct examination of skeletal muscle), NCV (examination of conduction along peripheral nerves) | Detection of myopathy, neuropathy, radiculopathy |
| Diagnostic nerve block: injection of a local anesthetic to determine the source and mechanism of the pain | Identification of structures responsible for the pain (eg, sacroiliac or facet joint blocks), differentiation of pain pathophysiology |

BUN, blood urea nitrogen; CBC, complete blood count; CNS, central nervous system; CSF, cerebrospinal fluid; CT, computed tomography; EMG, electromyography; ESR, erythrocyte sedimentation rate; MRI, magnetic resonance imaging; NCV, nerve conduction velocity; SCD, sickle cell disease; US, ultrasound

From Nonmalignant Pain in Palliative Medicine, by S. Weinstein, in D. Walsh, R. Fainsinger, K. Foley, et al. (Eds.), Palliative Medicine (Chapter 170, p. 934), 2009, Philadelphia: Saunders. © 2009 Elsevier. Reprinted with permission.

In some cases, changes in pain or associated manifestations over time may be necessary to clarify a differential diagnosis. This information may be obtained from a patient's history or a pain diary, which helps establish the pattern of painful episodes.[198] For example, important information can be obtained from a diary kept by a patient with chronic headache who develops metastatic disease. Stable recurrent episodes of headache do not require repeated evaluation, but a change in headache pattern may call for reimaging or examination of the cerebrospinal fluid. In a similar way, the assessment and management of low-back pain, joint pain, neuropathic pain states (eg, painful diabetic neuropathy, postherpetic neuralgia, nerve-injury related),[199,200] and other conditions such as fibromyalgia may require ongoing assessment of the pain pattern in the context of management strategies offered concurrently with treatments for the new illness.

# Pain Management

Treating chronic pain for patients with serious or life-threatening illness must be individualized, and the benefits, risks, and burdens related to the broader goals of palliation must be balanced. It is important to make a pain diagnosis and attempt to distinguish among chronic noncancer pain, acute or subacute cancer-related pain, and cancer pain associated with disease progression near the end of life. The treatment pathways may be quite different depending on the etiology of the pain. Specialist palliative care teams may be consulted when pain is difficult to control, is accompanied by other complex concerns, or occurs in the setting of advanced illness and short prognosis (the terminal care setting).[201] Some systems may have pain medicine specialists to help treat patients with refractory pain.

Treatment recommendations may include disease-modifying therapy, such as chemotherapy for sensitive cancers (eg, lymphoma, multiple myeloma, small cell lung cancer, ovarian cancer), and one or more types of pain-directed therapies, usually beginning with pharmacotherapy but also nonpharmacologic modalities (such as imagery, heat or cold therapies, music therapy, cognitive behavioral therapy, and spiritual counseling). This multimodal approach may focus on other symptoms (depression, anxiety, or demoralization) that impair analgesic responses and include communication, goal setting focused on function and not just reduction in pain intensity, care coordination, and family support. Patient education is an important component of pain management; patients need to understand the goals of therapy, what to anticipate from their illnesses and treatments, the proper use and possible side effects of medications, and safety concerns and behavioral expectations related to opioid prescriptions. Patients should have telephone numbers and access to clinicians who are guiding their pain management. Written material, educational brochures and handouts, and contact telephone numbers are critically important. Follow-up phone calls after outpatient visits can be helpful for assessing the effectiveness of the plan of care and reinforcing patient education.

Efforts to relieve pain are welcomed by patients, but such efforts fall short if the focus is largely on physical pain and not the whole person. Patients want efficient and effective measures taken to reduce pain but place a greater value on good clinicians who are willing to work as a team, listen to their story, communicate in a timely fashion, and show compassion.[2] Patients place as much value on how physicians care for them as they do for relief of their suffering.[2] Measuring pain is not difficult; it is determining what to do thereafter that is complex and difficult.

## Approach to Pain Management

Most cancer pain can be managed with relatively simple approaches; however, when pain is difficult to control, analgesic therapy may require complex pharmacotherapy or adjunctive strategies. The latter approaches may include a number of invasive procedures, which are generically labeled pain interventions.

## Treatment Considerations

The first step in developing a treatment strategy is to identify the etiology of the painful condition. Next, consider the feasibility, appropriateness, and potential effects of primary disease-modifying therapy. For example, in the setting of cancer pain, radiotherapy is commonly administered for analgesia and may be highly effective, particularly with bone lesions.[202] Although the literature on the potential analgesic effects of chemotherapy is complicated by methodological issues, the large number of regimens used, the limited availability of comparative trials, and other concerns,[203,204] the potential for pain-relieving effects may be one factor considered in decisions about the use of chemotherapy. Surgery is rarely indicated to treat cancer pain but may be considered in extreme circumstances. Palliative care clinicians should have a thorough understanding of the potential analgesic benefit of primary disease-modifying treatments for cancer pain.

In addition to disease-modifying therapy, most patients with persistent moderate or severe pain will require primary analgesic treatments. Pharmacotherapy is widely accepted as the main approach in the treatment of pain related to active, serious illness. Other treatment approaches are considered when drug therapy does not adequately control pain or is associated with intolerable adverse effects (see **Table 6**). Nondrug therapy may be particularly helpful in the management of chronic noncancer pain.[205,206]

## Pharmacologic Treatment

There are three main categories of drugs used to treat pain: nonopioid analgesics, which in the United States include nonsteroidal antiinflammatory drugs (NSAIDs) and acetaminophen; opioids; and an assortment of drug classes and agents referred to as adjuvant analgesics. Combination therapy with multiple analgesics is common in the treatment of chronic pain.

## World Health Organization Analgesic Ladder

Opioid-based pharmacotherapy has been viewed as the most important analgesic strategy for patients with life-threatening illness since the World Health Organization (WHO) posited the analgesic ladder approach for cancer pain more than 25 years ago (**Figure 5**).[207] The analgesic ladder is a simple framework for drug selection that incorporates guidelines for dose titration and other key aspects of treatment with opioids. Surveys suggest the approach can be used to provide effective pain relief for up to 90% of patients.[207]

The original analgesic ladder framework recommended a nonopioid for mild pain, a so-called weak opioid for moderate pain, and a so-called strong opioid for severe pain (see Figure 5). Nonopioid and other adjuvant analgesics could be added to opioids for steps 2 and 3. Also, step-2 analgesics have been bypassed with the use of low doses of potent opioids in countries where potent opioids are readily available.[208] The terms *weak* and *strong* have fallen out of favor. Also, a fourth step to the ladder has been suggested for instances in which traditional opioid and adjuvant analgesics do not provide adequate pain relief.[209] A broad array of approaches to drug selection and dosing includes the following:

## Table 6. Pain Treatment Categories[170]

| Category | Type of Treatment |
|---|---|
| Pharmacological | Opioid analgesics |
| | Nonopioid analgesics: acetaminophen, nonsteroidal anti-inflammatory drugs, topical agents, antidepressants, anticonvulsants, oral local anesthetics, steroids, cannabinoids, alpha-2 agonists, ketamine |
| Interventional | Spine or joint injection therapies |
| | Neurolytic blocks |
| | Spinal analgesics |
| | Surgical neuroablation |
| Rehabilitative | Physical modalities such as ultrasound |
| | Therapeutic exercise |
| | Occupational therapy |
| | Hydrotherapy |
| | Therapy for specific disorders such as lymphedema |
| | Heat/cold therapies |
| Psychological | Psychoeducational interventions |
| | Cognitive-behavioral therapy |
| | Relaxation therapy, guided imagery, other types of stress management |
| | Hypnotherapy |
| | Other forms of psychotherapy |
| Neurostimulation | Transcutaneous |
| | Transcranial |
| | Implanted (spinal or peripheral nerve) |
| Complementary/ Alternative or Integrative | Acupuncture |
| | Massage |
| | Physical/movement |
| | Music therapy |
| | Art therapy |
| | Other |

*Reprinted from* The Lancet, *377(9784), RK Portenoy, Treatment of Cancer Pain, 2236-2247, ©2011, with permission from Elsevier.*

## Figure 5. World Health Organization Cancer Pain Ladder

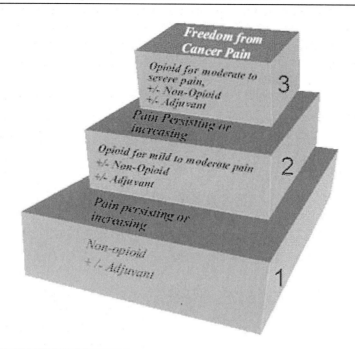

*Reprinted from* Cancer Pain Relief with a Guide to Opioid Availability, *2nd ed., 1996, Geneva, Switzerland: World Health Organization. © 1996 by World Health Organization.*

- Step 1. When pain is relatively mild, it may be sufficient to start with acetaminophen, an NSAID, or an adjuvant analgesic targeting a specific type of pain (eg, neuropathic, bone pain).
- Step 2. When pain persists, increases, or presents as mild to moderate, an opioid regimen should be considered. The choice may be an opioid conventionally used for moderate pain such as hydrocodone, a mixed-mechanism opioid (eg, tramadol, tapentadol), or a low starting dose of an opioid conventionally used for severe pain such as oxycodone or morphine. At Step 2, fixed-dosage combinations of an opioid with acetaminophen often are used because combining the drugs may provide added analgesia. When higher dosages of an opioid are needed, single-entity opioid and nonopioids are used to avoid toxic effects of high-dose acetaminophen and other NSAIDs. Adjuvant analgesics also are considered for specific types of pain. When Step 2 is initiated, medications for persistent pain are administered on an around-the-clock basis, with additional dosages as needed to control breakthrough pain.

- Step 3. When pain persists, increases, or initially presents as moderate to severe, single-entity, pure mu-agonist opioids are administered (eg, morphine, oxycodone, oxymorphone, hydromorphone, methadone, or fentanyl). Treatment will involve around-the-clock opioid administration for persistent pain, plus a supplemental short-acting drug as needed for breakthrough pain. Coadministration of acetaminophen or an adjuvant analgesic may be considered and added.
- Step 4. For chronic and unrelieved severe pain or intolerable opioid-related side effects, consider treatment with interventional techniques. Interventions include spinal analgesics, neurolytic blocks, spine steroid injections, and spinal cord stimulators.[210]

## The Science of Pain

 ### Opioid Receptors

There are three main opioid receptors—mu (MOR), delta (DOR), and kappa (KOR)—which are expressed as subtypes derived from splicing exon-derived mRNA involved in the transcription of receptor proteins. Four mu exons from the mu receptor gene are spliced into three classes of receptors, classified by the number of transmembrane domains in the protein transcribed. They include one (TM-1), six (TM-6 from exon 11 splicing in the gene promoter site), and seven (TM-7 derived from splicing of exon 4) transmembrane receptor proteins.[211] Each have a role in analgesia. Although there is only one mu gene, there is a large number of mu-receptor subtypes. Other opioid receptors such as the opioid-receptor-like orphan receptor (ORL-1) can be both analgesic and pronociceptive when activated by ligand nociception.[212,213] Sigma-1 receptors were considered at one time to be an opioid receptor because they were activated by certain opioids (pentazocine), but they are no longer considered opioid receptors. However, these receptors, which are normally located on endoplasmic reticulum near mitochondrion, when activated travel along the endoplasmic reticulum to interact with opioid receptors dampening G-protein activation and blunting opioid-induced analgesic responses. Haloperidol blocks sigma-1 receptor activation and in animal models improves the antinociception of morphine.

Opioid receptors are found on A delta and C afferent sensory neurons. Activation of opioid receptors inhibit presynaptic calcium channel peptide, thus preventing release of neurotransmitters such as glutamate, substance P, and calcitonin-gene related peptide. Opioids increase repolarization in postsynaptic neurons by activating potassium channels and inhibiting cyclic AMP production, resulting in hyperpolarization of second-order sensory neurons.

Opioids are classified as analgesics but more accurately are pain modulators that can both decrease and increase (opioid-induced hyperalgesia) the experience of pain.[214-218] Fortunately the overwhelming biologic effects opioids produce is analgesia. However, even when opioids act as analgesics, pain hypersensitivity to select stimuli can be detected by quantitative sensory testing. This includes increased sensitivity to cold stimulus, reduced tolerance to heat pain, increased temporal summation, and impaired conditioned pain modulation (which also is impaired in pain processing disorders such as fibromyalgia, diabetic neuropathy, and chemotherapy-induced neuropathy). Neuropathic pain is a hallmark of acute opioid withdrawal due to the sudden or abrupt discontinuation of opioids or administration of an opioid receptor antagonist such as naloxone to someone who has been taking opioids for a long time. Case reports of paradoxical pain with opioid titration are found in published literature.[219-221]

Certain opioid-related side effects (eg, immunosuppression, respiratory depression, hypogonadism, constipation, sleep-disordered breathing) are related to activation of opioid receptors, which are outside of the CNS pain matrix. Opioid receptors are expressed in a large number of non-neural tissues.[214] Endogenous opioids (eg, enkephalin, endorphins, endomorphins, dynorphin) do not have the same long-term side effects as exogenous opioids. For instance, endogenous opioids do not cause pain or hyperalgesia despite acting on the mu receptors. One reason for this is that endogenous opioids are regionally released, confined, and targeted to a specific site of action limiting "toxicity." Endogenous opioids are "short-acting" in nature.[222,223]

Opioids can cause pain by desensitizing mu receptors, upregulating NMDA receptors, and by increasing the function of NMDA receptors through phosphorylation of certain receptor subunits.[224] Brainstem periaqueductal gray/rostral ventromedial medulla (PAG/RVM) function facilitates rather than inhibits pain.[72] This neuroplastic brainstem response also is one of the mechanisms for neuropathic pain. Opioids cause neuroinflammation through activation of microglia and astrocytes. This occurs in a nonstereospecific fashion that does not require activation of opioid receptors. Opioids cause an increase in CNS interleukins and chemokines, which down-regulates opioid receptors and glutamate transporters, among other actions.[108,225-227] The end result of this neuroinflammatory response can be clinical depression, cognitive impairment, myoclonus, analgesic tolerance, and paradoxical pain. Neuroinflammation of a similar nature also is one of the hallmarks of neuropathic pain. Adjuvant analgesics such as gabapentinoids may improve the pain control of opioid therapy by blocking opioid pronociceptive responses.[228-233]

## Opioid Analgesics

The goal of long-term opioid therapy is to provide sustained, clinically meaningful relief of pain with tolerable side effects and an overall benefit to QOL. Guidelines, which are based on extensive international experience, limited evidence, and expert review,[169,207,234-237] provide a rationale for the selection of drug and route of administration, dosing, and side-effect management.[238-242]

### Drug Selection

Pure mu-agonist opioids conventionally are selected for pain treatment (**Table 7**). Important exceptions are meperidine and propoxyphene (no longer available in the United States), which are not recommended because of their potential for adverse effects, including myoclonus or seizures, especially for patients with renal dysfunction. Centrally acting drugs with mixed opioid-monoaminergic mechanisms such as tramadol and tapentadol may be used but have a ceiling due to risks for adverse events at higher doses, including seizures and serotonin syndrome; consequently, they offer less dosing flexibility. Although buprenorphine, a partial mu-receptor agonist and kappa-receptor antagonist, also may be used, pure mu-agonist drugs are preferred because experience with these drugs in medically ill patients is much more extensive. A recent systematic review suggests that buprenorphine could be considered as a fourth-line option for opioid treatment of cancer pain.[243]

The mixed agonist-antagonist opioids such as pentazocine and butorphanol offer little advantage and are not preferred in this setting. Combinations of oxycodone plus naloxone have been developed, both to reduce opioid-related constipation and to deter parenteral abuse.[244,245] Because oral naloxone is poorly bioavailable (less than 2%), there is little reversal of analgesia until doses over 120 mg a day are reached.[246] There is no advantage to using this agonist-antagonist combination for analgesia.

Other agonist-antagonist combinations have been developed for abuse deterrence and approved by the FDA (see https://www.fda.gov/Drugs/DrugSafety/InformationbyDrugClass/ucm337066.htm, Accessed August 1, 2017).[247-249] These agents should not be substituted for generic potent opioids unless there are clinical indications such as opioid-induced constipation refractory to standard laxatives or to prevent illicit route conversion of an opioid for someone at risk for misuse or abuse of opioids. In the United States, newer modified-release formulations such as long-acting oxycodone and morphine now include abuse-deterrent technology.[250] Opioid abuse–deterrent formulations either in market or under development also include hydrocodone, oxymorphone, tapentadol, and buprenorphine. These formulations incorporate either a mechanical or chemical strategy to reduce the likelihood that a tablet can be converted into an immediate-release opioid by crushing or dissolving. The objective is to benefit the public health by reducing the likelihood of abuse and unintentional overdose and possibly decreasing street market value to mitigate diversion. These benefits have not been established empirically; however, some clinical studies with recreational opioid abusers demonstrate reduced "drug liking" with the abuse-deterrent opioid formulations.[251,252]

## Table 7. Equianalgesic Table for Adults

| Opioid | Equianalgesic Doses (mg) | | Formulations Available |
| | Parenteral (SC/IV) | Oral | |
| --- | --- | --- | --- |
| Morphine | 10 | 30 | • IR oral tablet and capsule<br>• Oral solution (including concentrate)<br>• PR oral tablet and capsule<br>• Rectal suppository<br>• Parenteral |
| Buprenorphine | 0.3 | 0.4 (SL) | • Transmucosal tablet, buccal film<br>• Parenteral<br>• Transdermal patch |
| Codeine | 100 | 200 | • IR oral tablet<br>• Oral solution |
| Fentanyl | 0.1 | NA | • Transmucosal formulations<br>• Transdermal/iontophoretic<br>• Parenteral |
| Hydrocodone | NA | 30 | • IR oral tablet (in combination)<br>• PR oral tablet and capsule |
| Hydromorphone | 1.5 | 7.5 | • IR oral tablet<br>• Oral solution<br>• PR tablet<br>• Rectal suppository<br>• Parenteral |

**Table 7. Equianalgesic Table for Adults**

| Opioid | Equianalgesic Doses (mg) | | Formulations Available |
| | Parenteral (SC/IV) | Oral | |
|---|---|---|---|
| Meperidine (not recommended) | 100 | 300 | • IR oral tablet<br>• Oral solution<br>• Parenteral |
| Methadone | See notes | | |
| Oxycodone | 10* | 20 | • IR oral tablet and capsule<br>• Oral solution (including concentrate)<br>• PR oral tablet<br>• Parenteral* |
| Oxymorphone | 1 | 10 | • IR oral tablet<br>• PR oral tablet<br>• Parenteral |
| Tapentadol | NA | 100 | • IR oral tablet<br>• PR oral tablet |
| Tramadol | 100* | 120 | • IR oral tablet<br>• PR tablet and capsule<br>• Oral suspension<br>• Parenteral* |

*Not available in US

IR, immediate release; PR, prolonged release; SC, subcutaneous; SL, sublingual

Adapted from Demystifying Opioid Conversion Calculations: A Guide for Effective Dosing, by ML McPherson, Bethesda, MD: American Society of Health-System Pharmacists; 2010. © 2010 American Society of Health-System Pharmacists. Reprinted with permission.

Codeine and morphine were selected for the original WHO analgesic ladder, but there is no pharmacological rationale for this preference, particularly given the genetically determined variation in codeine's effects[253] and the potential influence of morphine metabolites on patients with renal impairment.[254] For patients with hepatic failure or severe liver disease, morphine and hydromorphone are preferred. For patients with renal failure or with significant impairment, methadone, fentanyl, or buprenorphine are preferred.[255-257] Because codeine requires conversion to morphine for analgesic effect, and some patients genetically may not be capable of this conversion, there is little rationale for the use of codeine to treat cancer or other chronic pain.

Cachexia delays oxycodone clearance, which means patients with cachexia should receive lower starting doses. On the other hand, cachexia is associated with decreased absorption of transdermal fentanyl, so higher doses may be required for effective pain relief.[258,259] For patients with significant weight loss,[260,261] experience with sequential opioid trials, or *opioid rotation*, highlights the importance of individual differences in response to various opioid drugs[262,263] and suggests that the most favorable opioid for an individual cannot be predicted. The important principle is that therapy may be initiated with any of the commonly used pure mu-agonist drugs, and clinicians should be prepared to switch, if necessary, to determine the drug that provides the best therapeutic outcomes.

The WHO analgesic ladder approach selects different opioids based on a moderate (eg, codeine) or severe (eg, morphine) pain intensity.[207] Although it remains common practice to follow this recommendation, any of the single-entity, pure mu-agonist drugs can be prescribed at dosages low enough to safely manage moderate pain, which eliminates the second "rung" of the ladder.[264]

Regular administration of an opioid to prevent or minimize chronic pain can be accomplished with a short- or long-acting opioid. In developed countries, long-acting drugs—either modified-release formulations (which have dosing intervals of 8 hours to 3 days) or a drug with a long half-life such as methadone generally are viewed as advantageous. They may increase convenience, reduce pill burden, and, at least theoretically, reduce the risk of a *bolus effect*—side effects at peak concentration or pain return at trough concentration. The ability to provide satisfactory relief with fixed-schedule dosages of a short-acting drug has been recognized for decades and remains an option in practice.

### Opioid Conversion Calculations

There are several reasons why a patient may need to be switched from one opioid, opioid route of administration, or opioid formulation to a different opioid regimen. These include poorly controlled pain, the development of an adverse effect, a change in patient status that requires a change in route of administration, formulary issues, drug shortages, or patient health beliefs that favor one opioid over another. Using equianalgesic conversion data (Table 7), prescribers can switch from one opioid regimen to another opioid regimen. The equivalency data shown in Table 7 is derived from studies of varying methodology; some are from single-dose studies, whereas others are comparisons done at steady state. Consequently, the equianalgesic dose table should be used only as a general guide.

It is important to follow a consistent process when performing an opioid conversion calculation. The following five-step process is recommended:[265]

1. Perform a comprehensive assessment of the patient's pain complaint. This serves two purposes. The first purpose is to determine if switching to a different opioid regimen is the most appropriate intervention as opposed to increasing the current opioid dose, adding a coanalgesic, or instituting a nonpharmacologic intervention. The second purpose is described in step 4—adjusting the newly calculated opioid regimen dose based on pain severity.

2. Determine the total daily opioid dose the patient is currently receiving. This includes the scheduled opioid dose and an average of the breakthrough opioid, if prescribed. If you do not have information about use of the rescue opioid, do not include it in the calculation of the average total daily dose.

3. Determine which opioid analgesic and route of administration the patient will be switched to, and set up a ratio based on data from the equianalgesic chart (Table 7).

4. After calculating an equivalent dose of the new opioid regimen, decide how to adjust the calculated dose based on data gathered from step 1. When switching to any opioid other than methadone or fentanyl, it is advisable to reduce the calculated dose by 25% to 50%—less reduction if the patient is still in pain, and a greater reduction if the patient is not in pain at the time of the switch. Considerations for conversion to methadone and fentanyl are discussed separately (see page 39).

5. The most important step of all is to carefully monitor the patient's response to the new opioid regimen. It may be necessary to implement a small dosage increase or decrease based on the patient's response to the new regimen.

## Clinical Situation

### Erald

Erald is a 68-year-old man admitted to hospice with a diagnosis of end-stage lung cancer with diffuse bony metastasis. He has comorbid conditions of diabetes mellitus, hypertension, dyslipidemia, and benign prostatic hyperplasia. On admission to hospice his medication regimen includes the following:

- Metformin, 1,000 mg by mouth twice a day
- Lisinopril, 20 mg by mouth once a day
- Atorvastatin, 40 mg by mouth once a day
- Tamsulosin, 0.4 mg by mouth once a day
- Finasteride, 5 mg by mouth once a day

- Morphine, 10 mg by mouth every 4 hours, as needed
- Diphenhydramine, 50 mg by mouth every 4 hours, as needed for itching
- Naproxen, 500 mg by mouth every 12 hours.

Erald states that when he takes four or five doses of the morphine in a 24-hour period, it adequately controls his pain. However, the morphine causes itching, for which his prescriber recommended diphenhydramine, 50 mg every 4 hours as needed. Unfortunately Erald states that when he takes the diphenhydramine he gets sleepy and feels like he's retaining urine. He also complains about having to take the morphine in the middle of the night, or he will awaken in significant pain. The prescriber decides to switch the patient from morphine, which should eliminate the need for diphenhydramine (which is causing adverse effects) to long-acting oxycodone. The following steps should be taken to convert Erald's morphine to oxycodone:

**Step 1.** An assessment of Erald's pain shows that the combination of morphine and naproxen adequately controls his pain and achieves his therapeutic goal. The reason for switching is twofold: to achieve a longer-lasting opioid effect and to relieve the adverse effect of pruritus.

**Step 2.** The patient keeps a log of morphine use, and the past 5 days show that he has consistently taken four or five doses of oral morphine, 10 mg per dose (40-50 mg oral morphine per day). It is safer to base the conversion calculation on the estimated 40 mg oral morphine per day.

**Step 3.** The prescriber has already decided to switch to oral long-acting oxycodone, but there are several other options for long-acting opioids (hydromorphone, hydrocodone, oxymorphone, methadone, tramadol, tapentadol). The equation below illustrates the calculation for switching from oral morphine to oral oxycodone. Always work in terms of total daily dose (TDD), as shown below:

$$\frac{X \text{ mg TDD oral oxycodone}}{40 \text{ mg TDD oral morphine}} = \frac{20 \text{ mg oral oxycodone}}{30 \text{ mg oral morphine}}$$

Cross multiply and solve for X as shown:

$$(x)(30) = (20)(40)$$

$$X = 26.7 \text{ mg oral oxycodone per day}$$

**Step 4.** In this step, individualize the calculated dose based on our knowledge of incomplete cross-tolerance when switching between opioids and the patient's current level of pain control. Because we are switching from one opioid to another, we should reduce the calculated dose by 25% to 50%. We calculated 26.7 mg oral oxycodone per day, therefore a 25% to 50% dose reduction gives us a potential dose range of 13.4 mg to 20 mg per day. The patient's pain is fairly well-controlled, so we could implement the greater dosage reduction, but the lowest tablet strength of long-acting oxycodone is 10 mg. Therefore, it would be appropriate to prescribe long-acting oxycodone, 10 mg orally every 12 hours. Because morphine causes an adverse effect (itching), we should use immediate release oxycodone for break-through pain. This is generally calculated as 10% to 15% of the total daily dose, or a low dose such as oxycodone, 5 mg orally every 2 hours as needed for additional pain.

**Step 5.** In the final step, we institute our new regimen and carefully observe the patient's response, both therapeutic and toxic. We will ask the patient to track his best, worst, and average pain rating daily as well as his use of the rescue oxycodone dose. When the patient is at steady-state (after 24-48 hours), we can increase the long-acting oxycodone if necessary. Of course, we would hold or reduce the dose if the patient experiences toxicity.

## Fentanyl and Methadone: Special Considerations
Expert panels designated transdermal fentanyl (TDF) and methadone as exceptions to the 30% to 50% equianalgesic dosage reduction to account for incomplete cross-tolerance, and each poses distinct challenges for dosing in general.[262,263]

### Transdermal Fentanyl
TDF may only be used for patients who are receiving at least 60 mg oral morphine daily, 30 mg oral oxycodone daily, 8 mg oral hydromorphone daily, or an equivalent dose of another opioid for at least a week. This precaution is in place due to the risk of respiratory depression. TDF may *not* be used for opioid-naïve patients.

The prescribing information for Duragesic (first TDF on the market) suggests the following conversion to TDF (**Table 8**). Please note that the table is not an equianalgesic table, and it only is recommended to covert to TDF, not from TDF to another drug.

The dosing guide in Table 8 is acknowledged to be very conservative. Many clinicians follow guidance provided by Breitbart and colleagues, as follows:[266]
- Calculate total daily dose of oral morphine (or calculate total daily dose of another opioid, not including methadone, and convert to oral morphine equivalent per day).
- Use a 2:1 ratio—every 2 mg oral morphine per day approximately equals 1 mcg per hour of TDF. For example, oral morphine 50 mg per day approximately equals TDF 25 mcg per hour.
- When the converted dosage falls between two different TDF patch strengths, round down to the closest available strength (25, 50, 75, 100 mcg/hour).

## Table 8. Converting from Morphine to Transdermal Fentanyl (Duragesic)

| Oral 24-hour morphine (mg/day) | Duragesic dose (mcg/hour) |
|---|---|
| 60-134 | 25 |
| 135-224 | 50 |
| 225-314 | 75 |
| 315-404 | 100 |
| 405-494 | 125 |
| 495-584 | 150 |
| 585-674 | 175 |
| 675-764 | 200 |
| 765-854 | 225 |
| 855-944 | 250 |
| 945-1,034 | 275 |
| 1,035-1,124 | 300 |

Fentanyl is a highly lipophilic opioid; it takes 12 to 24 hours for TDF to take full effect and 12 to 24 hours to dissipate after the patch is removed. TDF is applied for continuous administration and is usually dosed every 72 hours; a small percentage of patients require dosing every 48 hours.

A transdermal system, such as TDF, is not an optimal drug delivery system for patients with a rapidly changing pain presentation. Release of fentanyl from a transdermal system may be accelerated if the patient becomes febrile or local heat is applied over the patch area. Clinicians have observed a suboptimal response to TDF for patients who are cachectic. If this is suspected, be very conservative when switching off TDF (in other words, do not assume the patient was fully absorbing the fentanyl from the transdermal patch).

Transmucosal Immediate Release Fentanyl (TIRF) has been formulated to include oral transmucosal lozenge, buccal tablet, sublingual tablet, sublingual spray, buccal soluble film, and nasal spray. Use of TIRF is restricted to opioid-tolerant cancer patients only. Opioid tolerance is defined as use of at least 60 mg of oral morphine (or equivalent) for 1 week or longer. Use requires participation in the Risk Evaluation and Mitigation Strategy (REMS) Access program (https://www.tirfremsaccess.com/TirfUI/rems/home.action). This program requires the registration of prescribers and pharmacies as well as patients who are prescribed a TIRF.

TIRF includes sublingual, intranasal, and buccal administration. Preparations are expensive and have unique properties with which prescribers should become familiar before prescribing.

Rules for prescribing TIRFs as a breakthrough medication should not be considered the same as for other opioids in terms of the ratio between the total daily dosage and the breakthrough dose. Furthermore, all TIRFs have a black box warning that states practitioners should not convert patients to TIRF products from another product, or among TIRF products. Always start at the lowest dose and titrate per the manufacturer's directions (which vary between all six products). TIRFs have an immediate onset of action within minutes and duration of action of 1 to 2 hours.

## Methadone

Rotation to methadone raises specific challenges and deserves additional comment. Methadone-associated risk has been receiving increasing scrutiny in populations with chronic non-cancer pain, and the lessons learned should be translated to medically ill patients.[267] As noted, methadone often is considered when a high dose of another opioid results in unacceptable side effects.[268] In addition to its opioid agonist activity, methadone blocks the NMDA receptor, which may contribute to analgesia and reverse a component of opioid analgesic tolerance.[268] Presumably, as a consequence, methadone has a poorly predictable potency when administered after another opioid has been taken—its potency generally will be much greater if started after relatively high doses of another opioid have been taken. The potential for enhanced and unpredictable potency after a switch from any other opioid to methadone poses a risk for unintentional overdose and has justified the recommendation that rotation to methadone be accompanied by a large reduction in the calculated equianalgesic dose.[263] The half-life of methadone averages about 24 hours but is highly variable, ranging from half a day to almost 1 week. This variability imposes additional risk. With steady-state levels in blood approached after five to six half-lives, effects must be monitored for a relatively long period after the dose is changed to anticipate the relatively long period required to be at steady state.

Several additional potential risks are associated with methadone. Given its metabolism by the cytochrome P450 system, drug-drug interactions are possible, particularly with drugs metabolized by CYP3A4.[269] Equally important, it is now appreciated that methadone prolongs the corrected QT (QTc) interval, and knowledge of the baseline QTc and monitoring as methadone doses are increased may be needed to optimize safety, particularly in the setting of polypharmacy to address multiple disorders.[270-272]

In short, despite strong analgesic potential, good oral bioavailability (80%), and relatively stable kinetics in renal impairment, methadone has both unique pharmacokinetic and pharmacodynamic characteristics that may increase risk and must be understood to provide safe and effective therapy.[273,274] The potential for highly favorable outcomes has been suggested in observational studies, and although controlled trials have not been able to confirm this benefit, continued reliance on methadone is likely given clinical experience, its long dosing interval, flexibility of multiple routes of administration, and low cost.[275-278] Its concurrent use as a treatment for opioid craving for those with addiction also suggests that it may have value when patients with substance use disorders develop pain. If a patient has an active substance use disorder, however, the complexity of management may be best addressed with the help of a specialist in addiction medicine.

Given the risks associated with methadone, a 2014 consensus document suggested specific guidelines for rotating to this drug.[279] Specifically, a switch to methadone from another opioid should be accompanied by a large reduction in the calculated equianalgesic dose. A decrease of 75% to 90% has been recommended; reductions near the upper bound of this range should be used when the switch is in the context of high-dose prior therapy or when patients are medically frail. A second-step dose change of up to 15% can be considered thereafter to accommodate more risk (eg, a dose reduction if there is a coadministered benzodiazepine) or severe pain (a dose increase). A panel of hospice and palliative medicine experts further developed recommendations for switching to methadone, either as a 10:1 or 20:1 conversion from oral morphine (**Table 9**). Experts recommend converting to methadone at no more than 30 mg to 40 mg per day regardless of the previous opioid regimen.[279]

Additional precautions should be observed: Treatment with methadone should be preceded by review of a baseline QTc interval in most cases. An interval of 500 milliseconds or longer should be considered an absolute contraindication to methadone therapy, and an interval longer than 450 milliseconds should be considered a relative contraindication and prompt an effort to remove other contributing factors to QTc prolongation (eg, another drug), if possible.[279] Unless the goals of care are such that monitoring is not appropriate, repeated electrocardiograms (ECGs) during dose escalation must be considered, although a prospective trial did not conclude this intervention was essential for patients with cancer.[270,279] Monitoring a patient's reaction to methadone should be frequent after therapy is initiated or the dose is increased; monitoring should become routine only when clinical stability has suggested steady-state levels. Methadone's risk profile is such that it is best used cautiously when other sedating centrally acting drugs are being administered, particularly benzodiazepines. Combination with benzodiazepines anecdotally has been linked with an increased risk of opioid-induced sleep disordered breathing.

## Tips for Safe Methadone Dosing

The long and variable half-life of methadone (6-190 hours) can lead to drug accumulation, sedation, confusion, and respiratory depression, especially in older people or with rapid dose adjustments.[280]

Because of the long half-life of methadone, the rapid titration guidelines used for other opioids do not apply to methadone. Dose-conversion ratios are complex and vary based on current opioid dosage and patient-specific factors.

Because of the potential for drug accumulation from the long half-life, always write "hold for sedation" when initially prescribing or changing dosages of methadone.

Methadone in moderate to high dosages can prolong the QTc interval and increase the risk of the potentially lethal torsades de pointes arrhythmia. Depending on goals of treatment, presence of associated heart disease, the patient's prognosis, presence of other medications that might cause similar problems (eg, haloperidol), or presence of new QTc prolongation risk factors, consider checking the QTc at baseline, and begin monitoring it after each dose change

## Table 9. Conversion from Morphine to Methadone

| Oral morphine equivalent/24 hours | Suggested conversion to methadone |
|---|---|
| Up to 60 mg | Not to exceed methadone 2.5 mg PO every 8 hours |
| 60 mg-199 mg | Use a 10:1 (oral morphine in 24 hours to oral methadone in 24 hours) ratio (do not exceed 30 mg as a total daily starting dose) |
| 200 mg or higher (and in older adults and vulnerable patients) | Use a 20:1 (oral morphine in 24 hours to oral methadone in 24 hours) ratio (do not exceed 30 mg as a total daily starting dose) |

for patients taking more than 100 mg of methadone daily. If QTc prior to starting methadone or during methadone therapy is between 450 and 500 milliseconds, consider an alternative to methadone. If the QTc interval is 500 milliseconds or greater at any time, guidelines recommend against the use of methadone. Consider formal consultation with palliative care, acute pain service, cardiology, and pharmacy.

Medications that can decrease methadone levels include rifampin, phenytoin, corticosteroids, carbamazepine, bosentan, phenobarbital, St. John's Wort, and a number of antiretroviral agents.

Medications that can increase methadone levels include tricyclic antidepressants, azole antifungals (especially voriconazole), macrolides and fluoroquinolones, amiodarone, selective serotonin reuptake inhibitors (SSRIs), and diazepam. Grapefruit juice also can increase methadone levels. Consider reducing calculated dosages of methadone by 25% to 30%.

Methadone is best used as a baseline, scheduled analgesic, with shorter-acting opioids such as morphine or hydromorphone used as needed for breakthrough pain. The dose for this rescue opioid should be 10% to 15% of the previous nonmethadone regimen (eg, if the prior regimen was morphine sulfate controlled release [MS Contin], 60 mg by mouth every 12 hours, the breakthrough dose should be short-acting morphine, 10 mg or 15 mg by mouth every 2 hours as needed). If the patient is opioid naive, start a short-acting rescue opioid at a customary starting dosage (eg, morphine, 5 mg by mouth every 2 hours as needed).

In stable situations with excellent patient compliance, small doses of methadone can be given as needed in addition to the scheduled regimen, but never more than 2.5 mg to 5 mg two or three times daily. Small incremental doses in patients receiving a large baseline dose may have a major effect on blood level if taken regularly.

For patients who are opioid naïve, or those regularly receiving up to 40 mg to 60 mg oral morphine equivalent per day, begin methadone no higher than 2.5 mg by mouth three times daily. Consider very low doses for vulnerable patients (eg, 1 mg by mouth every 12 hours).

When converting from more than 60 mg oral morphine equivalent per day, the American Pain Society guidelines recommend "75% to 90% less than calculated equianalgesic dose."[280] When converting from oral to intravenous methadone, reduce the total daily dose of methadone by 50%. When converting from intravenous methadone to oral methadone, use 1:1 conversion to avoid overmedicating the patient; carefully observe the patient for under- and overdosing. Always consider potential drug interactions and adjust accordingly.

## Drugs for Breakthrough Pain

Breakthrough pain (**Table 10**) has been reported in 40% to 80% of patients with cancer, depending on the clinical setting.[296,297] With growing recognition of the negative consequences resulting from breakthrough pain,[281] a short-acting drug is usually offered as needed during regular opioid treatment. Depending on the opioid dose required and other factors, this rescue drug may be an opioid-non-opioid combination product, a single-entity oral opioid such as morphine or oxycodone, or a rapid-onset fentanyl formulation.

These supplemental opioid doses for breakthrough pain variably are called *rescue doses, breakthrough doses,* or *escape doses.* If an oral formulation is used, the dose usually is 10% to 15% of the baseline daily dose prescribed every 1 to 2 hours. For example, a patient receiving modified-release morphine at a dose of 100 mg every 12 hours (100 mg × 2 doses = 200 mg daily) may be prescribed a rescue dose of 20 mg to 30 mg every 1 to 2 hours. Choice may be limited by what formulations are commercially available; for example, short-acting morphine tablets are not available in a 20 mg dose in the United States. For patients receiving an opioid infusion, a dose equal to 50% to 100% of the hourly infusion rate every 10 to 15 minutes can be used. For example, a patient receiving a hydromorphone infusion at 1 mg/hour may be offered a rescue dose of 0.5 mg to 1 mg every 10 to 15 minutes. The safety of this proportionate dosing has not been established for rapid-onset fentanyl formulations, and treatment with these drugs should start with the lowest or next-to-lowest dose strength.[282]

## Table 10. Types of Breakthrough Pain

| Type | Characteristics | Pharmacologic Strategies |
| --- | --- | --- |
| Incident | Activity-related<br>Has identifiable precipitant | Use a short-acting rescue dose if possible; anticipate and premedicate with a short-acting agent; optimize the baseline regimen. |
| Idiopathic/spontaneous | Unpredictable | Use a short-acting rescue dose if possible; optimize the baseline regimen. |
| End-of-dose failure | Predictable return of pain before next scheduled dose of medication | Increase the dose or shorten the time between doses of the baseline regimen or, if necessary, use a short-acting rescue dose. |

In all cases titration of the rescue dose may be needed to optimize the balance between analgesia and side effects. If a rescue dose is needed three or more times daily, this may signal the need to increase the baseline dose or change the analgesic strategy.

The rapid-onset fentanyl formulations were developed to address the evident mismatch between the time course of breakthrough pain (which typically peaks within minutes and lasts less than 1 hour) and the time-action relationship of an oral drug (which starts to work at 30 to 45 minutes and peaks after 1 hour). All of these formulations, which now include an oral transmucosal lozenge, an effervescent buccal tablet, a buccal patch, a sublingual tablet, and nasal sprays, provide a means for a highly lipophilic opioid to enter the bloodstream quickly via the transmucosal route. Clinical observations and limited comparative trials[283] suggest that the rapid-onset formulations yield faster pain relief and better outcomes, at least for some patients.[284,285] Although further study will be needed to assess the safety of these drugs and optimally position them relative to oral agents, it is reasonable to consider them for patients with severe breakthrough pain that peaks quickly, for those who do not respond well to oral drugs, and for patients lacking availability of the oral route.

## Routes of Administration

The oral and transdermal routes of administration are preferred for long-term management of pain. The intramuscular route is not used because it is painful and provides no pharmacological advantage. Alternative routes of administration are considered in select circumstances. One can consider the use of intravenous infusions versus subcutaneous routes in less intensive settings. Almost all opioids can be given subcutaneously except methadone, which causes skin toxicity. Home or facility parenteral infusions or patient-controlled analgesia (PCA) may be necessary for patients on high-dose opioids or who cannot swallow and do not have a percutaneous gastric tube. Hydromorphone in particular can be highly concentrated. Alternative long-acting sublingual opioids methadone and buprenorphine could be used. Many patients have central ports, midlines, or percutaneous-placed central catheters that can be used for parenteral opioids in lieu of SC-placed lines.[286,287] Most sustained-release opioids and immediate-release opioids are absorbed per rectum and can be used in an emergency.[287,288]

## Clinical Situation

### Salim

Salim is a 45-year-old man with laryngeal cancer who had major head and neck surgery, including resection and reconstruction. He is undergoing chemotherapy and radiation therapy and has severe mouth and neck pain, along with painful mucositis. He is no longer able to swallow and receives all of his nutrition and medication through a percutaneous endoscopic gastrostomy (PEG) tube. His current analgesics are oxycodone extended release, 15 mg every 12 hours, with immediate release oxycodone, 5 mg for breakthrough pain. He currently crushes all of his medications and takes them through the PEG tube.

**?** What are the major issues for pain management you see in this case?

**?** Should he be screened for risk of addiction?

**?** Should you educate him about expectations around safe use and monitor him for aberrant drug-taking behaviors?

**?** What instructions would you give to this patient?

**?** What opioids can be crushed and given through a PEG tube? What opioids should not be crushed for administration?

**?** What sustained-release opioid can be given through his PEG?

**?** Are there some alternative routes of administration that would be more appropriate?

**?** What regimen would you recommend for treatment of the mucositis pain?

Salim likely has neuropathic pain secondary to cancer treatment. Tobacco and alcohol abuse are major risk factors for laryngeal cancer. A thorough drug and alcohol history is warranted to assess the risk for addiction. Even though he has cancer pain that would be excluded from the CDC guideline for prescribing opioids for chronic pain,[27] he should be educated about expectations for safe use and monitored for aberrant drug-taking behaviors. The patient should be given detailed instructions on when he should take his medication, how much, and how often he can use a breakthrough dose. He should be cautioned about not taking more than prescribed, and he should be given telephone numbers and names of case managers and physicians to contact if his pain is poorly controlled or he has side effects. A general educational handout on opioids that also contains particulars about side effects should be provided. He should be instructed to not share his opioid with family members or friends, and he should keep his opioid in a safe place, preferably locked away in a safe or locked cabinet. Sustained-release opioids should not be crushed and placed in a PEG. Certain sustained-release opioids come as pellets within a capsule which can be opened and given through a PEG followed by a water or saline flush. Other long-acting alternatives include methadone, which can be given as a liquid, or buprenorphine, which can be given sublingually. There are no standard medications for mucositis approved by the US Food and Drug Administration (FDA). Analgesics, mouth rinses, and topical analgesics have been used to manage mucositis.

## Transdermal Administration

Although most clinicians consider the oral route first, some patients prefer transdermal administration, some benefit from access to fentanyl specifically, and some have problems with swallowing or gastrointestinal (GI) absorption that may be addressed through nonoral drug administration.[289] Transdermal and sublingual absorption of opioids are directly related to the lipophilicity of the particular opioid. Lipophilicity is determined by the relative affinity of a substance to partition into a layer of octanol (a fatty alcohol) or into water—the higher the lipophilicity, the greater the ability to cross mucous membranes and skin.[290] Several studies suggest the transdermal fentanyl formulation is associated with less constipation,[291] and this may be another reason to use transdermal opioids. Also, fentanyl transdermal absorption is reduced among patients with cachexia, but intravenous fentanyl plasma levels are increased. Clinically, pain control may be lost when converting parenteral fentanyl to transdermal fentanyl for patients who are suffering from cachexia.[258,259] Aluminum-containing backing to fentanyl transdermal patches may cause a burn to patients who are undergoing a magnetic resonance imaging (MRI) procedure.[292] Buprenorphine transdermal patches may be used as an alternative, although doses are limited to no more than 20 mcg per hour in the United States. Patches are changed weekly.

When initiating treatment with the transdermal fentanyl formulation, the equianalgesic dose table from the package insert may be used to select a starting dose. The dose ratios built into this table are conservative, and most patients will require dose escalation to experience pain relief. A simple alternative method of initial dose selection is to divide the 24-hour total dose of oral morphine by two to get a starting dose of transdermal fentanyl. For example,[293] a patient taking 400 mg of oral morphine in 24 hours would be switched to 200 mcg per hour of transdermal fentanyl every 72 hours.

Like other long-acting drugs, transdermal fentanyl should not be used to rapidly titrate the dose when pain is severe. In most situations the dose should not be titrated upward more frequently than every 72 hours. Because clinically relevant plasma fentanyl concentrations do not occur for 12 to 24 hours after the initial dose is applied, patients should be continued on their previous drugs for this period following a switch to transdermal fentanyl.[294] The administration of a short-acting rescue opioid also provides a means to avoid uncontrolled pain during initial titration.

The risks associated with transdermal fentanyl are similar to risks associated with all opioids, with a few exceptions such as skin hypersensitivity. The most important difference is the risk of unintentional overdose from increased absorption associated with heat, either due to fever or an external heat source. As a result of this concern, the patch is not recommended for patients with recurrent fever. Also, reduced fentanyl absorption may occur among patients with cachexia.

Transdermal buprenorphine also has been used in the treatment of chronic noncancer or cancer pain. The patch is applied to the upper body similar to fentanyl. Following application, plasma levels increase over the next 2 days, and the patch is changed every week. An advantage to buprenorphine for older patients is that pharmacokinetics are unchanged with age and with renal failure. Transdermal buprenorphine is available in the United States in 5-, 7.5-, 10-, 15-, and 20-mcg per hour formulations.[295,296]

### Sublingual Administration
Occasionally the sublingual route of administration is considered for patients who lose the ability to swallow. The lipophilic opioids such as fentanyl, methadone, and buprenorphine are absorbed through the oral mucosa relatively well.[297] Sublingual administration of the injectable fentanyl has been reported to be effective and is relatively inexpensive, if the dose requirements are relatively low. Methadone may be considered if guidelines for safe administration are followed (see Opioid Rotation on page 59). Sublingual buprenorphine can induce opioid withdrawal if administered to patients on methadone doses greater than 45 mg per day or morphine doses greater than 120 mg per day. Consequently it should only be used by knowledgeable clinicians experienced in its administration. For patients on buprenorphine, other immediate-release oral formulations such as morphine, oxycodone, or hydromorphone can be given for breakthrough pain.[298,299] When hydrophilic opioids like morphine are given sublingually, they are absorbed mostly after being swallowed and not mucosally.

### Rectal Administration
A variety of opioids and adjuvant medications can be administered rectally in suppository form (see Table 7). Slow-release morphine tablets inserted into an empty, moist rectum can deliver 12 hours of analgesia, comparable to oral administration.[300] Custom-made methadone suppositories have proved effective in a wide range of dosages.[301,302] A number of adjuvant analgesics such as naproxen can be administered rectally by instilling the oral solution into the rectum using an enema bulb, urinary catheter, or a 6-inch length of nasal-prong oxygen tubing attached to a syringe. Some drugs, such as doxepin, come in gelatin capsules that dissolve in the rectum. Others can be crushed and put into large gel capsules for rectal insertion.[303]

Rectal administration is associated with variable absorption because of variation in venous drainage, placement of the suppository, and contents of the rectum. Long-term administration in sentient patients is rarely acceptable. Accordingly, rectal administration is usually considered for short-term drug administration, perhaps for actively dying patients or as an interim step during the transition from oral to long-term parenteral administration.

## Parenteral Administration

Patients who may benefit from parenteral drug administration include those with dysphagia, persistent nausea, and vomiting. Patients receiving high dosages of oral opioids that require numerous tablets also are good candidates. Long-term intravenous or subcutaneous drugs are delivered as repeated boluses or infusions. With widespread access to syringe drivers or computer-activated delivery device (CADD) pumps in developed countries, infusions are a common practice.

Patients who already have an indwelling central venous catheter will generally be treated with intravenous rather than subcutaneous therapy unless there are extenuating circumstances, such as ongoing parenteral nutrition. The advent of peripherally inserted central catheters (PICCs) has expanded the use of intravenous delivery of opioid therapy. These catheters are placed with minimal patient burden and may be used for home delivery of opioid therapy.[304] Placement of PICC lines should be confirmed by chest X ray.

Subcutaneous therapy is a simple alternative to the intravenous route and is the more common practice internationally. Subcutaneous lines can use a 21-gauge butterfly catheter and small-gauge needle inserted under the skin and can be left in place for 1 week or sometimes longer. This catheter can be accessed for repeated boluses or connected to a pump for continuous subcutaneous infusion. Any opioid or combination of opioid and adjuvant drugs (eg, opioid plus antiemetic such as metoclopramide or haloperidol) available in injectable formulations can be administered in this way.[305] However, subcutaneous methadone is painful and will produce nodules during subcutaneous dosing. Morphine and hydromorphone are the most common opioids selected for continuous infusion. Hydromorphone dose concentrations can be as high as 50 mg/mL, and because of morphine's limited solubility, is a preferred choice for high-dose opioid subcutaneous infusions. Commercial hydromorphone solutions in 10 mg/mL are available, but if the dose requirement is high, a more concentrated solution (50 mg/mL) can be mixed from powder.

Hydration by the subcutaneous route (known as hypodermoclysis) is a technique that can be combined with palliative drug delivery (eg, haloperidol, opioids, metoclopramide). Hyaluronidase may be added to the infusate to facilitate absorption of subcutaneous infusions.

To switch from an oral opioid to the intravenous or subcutaneous route of the same drug, the dose of the parenteral drug should be selected using the equianalgesic dose table (Table 7). The oral bioavailability of the opioid largely dictates the conversion ratio. Oral bioavailability of morphine is 30%, so the conversion from oral to subcutaneous or intravenous morphine is 3:1. Dose adjustments will need to be made based on analgesia and toxicity after route conversion. If converting from a sustained-release opioid such as sustained-release morphine, parenteral doses should be started at a lower than equianalgesic dose unless they are delayed and started only after the sustained-release dose is wearing off (Table 7).

Patients receiving parenteral opioids for pain are offered a supplemental rescue dose for breakthrough pain. PCA options often are used, but the patient must have requisite cognitive and physical abilities to operate the device and be willing to do so.[306] The rescue dose during parenteral infusion is usually proportional to the infused dose—50% to 100% of the amount administered over a 1-hour period. There are a large number of different PCA strategies that are used clinically, with demand dose lock-out intervals ranging from 10 to 60 minutes. There are no randomized trials that clarify which dose and interval is optimal. The strategy may require adaptation to the patient's pain pattern, including the temporal nature of the pain as well as pain severity and type of breakthrough pain. Incident pain may require a higher rescue dose. This rescue dose interval varies widely among clinicians. Lock-out intervals range from every 10 to 15 minutes to once hourly as needed. There are no randomized trials to guide the practice. Some patients will repeatedly activate the device to prevent pain from coming back. Some patients whose continuous opioid dose is suboptimal may frequently activate the device to maintain pain control but will experience pain early in the morning because they did not activate the PCA throughout the night. Methadone can be delivered by continuous infusion but should not be combined with an as-needed rescue dose.

The concept that three boluses or more needed during the day means that the around-the-clock dose should be increased needs to be interpreted with caution. Many people treated with a PCA will have reduced pain in the postoperative setting or with procedures (eg, surgery, single fraction radiation). Another group will have incident pain, which only occurs with movement even though baseline pain is well-controlled. If these patients become active, they may frequently activate the PCA for incident pain but have stable baseline pain. Increasing the around-the-clock dosage would lead to opioid toxicity between periods of activity. Titration of the baseline parenteral dose should not be done more than once per day, and adjustment of the around-the-clock dosage should only be done when it has reached steady state (usually 20 to 24 hours or 4 to 5 drug half-lives). Pain that recurs before then should be managed by increasing the rescue dose by 50% to 100% (25% for frail patients and those with organ failure).

Patients must be monitored while on a PCA. It is a mistake to believe that the lock-out mechanism will prevent opioid overdose. Patients should only be on as-needed doses by PCA rather than infusion if they only have episodic pain. This sometimes is done when patients are on transdermal fentanyl for continuous pain that is controlled but who are experiencing intermittent acute pain from a procedure or breakthrough pain. A PCA demand-only strategy has also been used on the first day or two of opioid therapy to gauge the needs of the patient before starting around-the-clock dosages. This is a reasonable strategy to use if a patient is unstable or developing significant organ failure, which would influence the clearance of the opioid. This also may be considered for patients who are relatively opioid naive. The best approach for patients who require rapid titration for severe pain is clinician-based bedside opioid titration to acceptable analgesia using small, frequent doses of morphine, hydromorphone, or fentanyl followed by placing the patient on a PCA with the continuous dose based on the effective titrated opioid dose and a proportional rescue dose. The initial dose finding with the PCA alone may enable a more informed selection of the infusion rate. The most important part of delivering opioids by a PCA is to frequently reassess the patient; do not "set and forget."

## Percutaneous Gastric Tube Administration

Morphine sulfate and naltrexone hydrochloride extended release capsules (Embeda), indicated for the management of chronic, moderate to severe pain, contain extended-release morphine pellets with a sequestered naltrexone core. The capsule can be opened and the pellets administered through a percutaneous endoscopic gastrostomy (PEG) tube. Morphine sulfate extended-release capsules (Kadian) also come in pellet form.[307] The capsule can be opened and pellets given through a PEG tube without loss of the extended-release pharmacokinetics. Methadone tablets can be crushed or the oral elixir given via the PEG tube as another long-acting opioid. Most immediate release non–tamper resistant opioids and elixirs can be given through a PEG tube. The tablets will need to be crushed.

## Neuraxial Drug Administration

Properly selected patients can benefit from spinal analgesic therapy, known generically as neuraxial infusion.[308] A randomized trial comparing conventional analgesic therapy and neuraxial infusion via an implanted programmable pump in patients with cancer found that neuraxial infusion yielded better analgesia and fewer side effects.[309] If this option is available, it should be considered among a range of strategies for patients with pain refractory to routine systemic therapy.

The best indication for a trial of neuraxial infusion is when a patient experiences meaningful pain relief during systemic therapy with an opioid but is unable to tolerate the side effects. In this situation, many options may be considered, presumably the most common of which is opioid rotation. Neuraxial analgesia is another strategy.[310,311]

Neuraxial analgesia may be provided through either the epidural or subarachnoid (intrathecal) route. Epidural drug administration may be accomplished using a percutaneous catheter (either anchored to the back or tunneled subcutaneously and emerging anteriorly) or a catheter that is tunneled and connected to an implanted port. The former route is simpler to implement but less durable and more subject to infection and technical problems such as catheter dislodgement. For patients with a perceived life expectancy of more than 3 months and for those with pathology that complicates placement of an epidural catheter, such as vertebral compression fractures or radiation-induced fibrosis,[310] the intrathecal route is preferred. Based on limited data, it is generally accepted that the cumulative costs of an implanted system are lower than for an epidural system if the patient has a life expectancy of 3 months or longer.

Intrathecal delivery devices should be implanted and maintained by providers trained and skilled specifically in intrathecal drug delivery. Clinicians must be fully aware of prescribing information for all devices and drugs used in the devices. Successful therapy requires a partnership in which the patient takes responsibility for adherence to physician recommendations, self-monitoring, and vigilance for adverse effects.[312] Educating patients and families is of utmost importance. Respiratory depression is the key therapy-related safety issue with spinal analgesia. Respiratory depression is defined as a reduced respiratory rate (less than 10 to 12 breaths per minute); reduced oxygen saturation (arterial oxygen saturation less than 90% to

92%); hypercapnia (arterial $CO_2$ retention greater than 50 mm Hg); or clinical signs of drowsiness, sedation, periodic apnea, and/or cyanosis.[313] Deaths associated with spinal analgesia are related to clinicians prescribing oral or parenteral sedatives, hypnotics, opioids, antidepressants, and/or antihistaminics to patients undergoing spinal analgesia. Therefore, a single provider should supervise all of the patient's CNS-active medications while the patient is receiving spinal analgesia.[312]

## Spinal Opioid Pharmacology

There is a magnitude of difference between cerebrospinal fluid (CSF) production (1 mL per 30 seconds) and flow rate (40 mcL per day). CSF moves mostly in an oscillating (to and fro) manner, more so in the cervical than the lumbar spine area and not by CSF bulk flow.[314,315] Recent findings suggest that drug distribution within the CSF is limited to a few centimeters and does not disperse completely around the spinal cord.[316] The main generator that causes dispersion of CSF oscillation is associated with alternating systole and diastole. Paradoxically, delivering the same dose of drug at higher flow rates rather than increasing the concentration and maintaining the flow rate does not improve response but increases adverse effects and reduces QOL.[317,318] This is the rationale behind changing drug concentrations rather than increasing infusion rates when titrating spinal analgesics.

The relative potency of opioids in the epidural and intrathecal spaces is largely dependent on the lipophilic character of the particular opioid. Spinal availability of epidural opioids is dependent on the redistribution of the opioid from the epidural space into the spinal cord.[319] There is a strong linear relationship between lipid solubility and the mean resident time of an opioid. The more lipid-soluble opioids spend greater time in the epidural space and sequestered in fat, with less ability to migrate into the CSF. As a result, epidural fentanyl and sufentanil have a lower intrathecal area-under-the-curve distribution. Epidural-sequestered fentanyl and sufentanil are released back into circulation. Plasma concentrations from epidural injection or infusion of both lipophilic opioids are equivalent to the same dose using parenteral infusions. Intrathecal opioid pharmacokinetics and distribution also determine the relative potency of opioids. Because permeability through meninges favors moderately lipophilic opioids, they have a much greater volume of distribution relative to hydrophilic opioids such as morphine (40 times greater). This is due to rapid partitioning of intrathecal lipophilic opioids to epidural fat and spinal white matter away from gray matter, where sensory neurons and opioid receptors reside. As a result, the analgesia of intrathecal lipophilic opioids is partly dependent upon systemic absorption. For both intrathecal and epidural analgesic administration, it is important for the analgesic catheter tip to be in close proximity to the spinal cord level at which nociception is occurring.

In contrast, morphine concentrates in spinal extracellular fluid around the superficial dorsal horn sensory neurons within the gray matter to a dramatically greater degree than lipophilic opioids.[321] By parenteral injection, 10 mg of morphine is equivalent to 10 mcg of sufentanil. However, by intrathecal injection, 10 mcg of sufentanil is equivalent to only 100 mcg of morphine, a 100-fold difference. In the same manner, by parenteral injection fentanyl is 100-fold more potent than morphine, but by intrathecal injection fentanyl is only 2 to 4 times more potent than morphine, a 25-fold difference.[322]

Morphine is the most spinal-selective opioid used for intrathecal and epidural analgesia (**Table 11**). The normal conversion ratio for oral morphine to epidural morphine is 10:1 and from oral morphine to intrathecal morphine is 100:1. Early analgesia from spinal morphine is related to selective actions within the superficial dorsal horn. Late analgesia is by way of CSF rostral spread to brainstem sites.[322] The slow rostral migration or redistribution of morphine to the brainstem also accounts for the delayed respiratory depression that can be seen with spinal morphine therapy.

**Neuraxial Adjuvant Analgesics**
**Local Anesthetics.** Lidocaine is hydrophilic and poorly protein bound. Lidocaine gains rapid access to the superficial dorsal horn and has a medium duration of analgesic response. It can cause transient pain in the gluteal region and lower extremities, as can other local anesthetics. This occurs more frequently with lidocaine than with other local anesthetics. Lidocaine has been superseded by levobupivacaine, bupivacaine, and ropivacaine.[323] Local anesthetics can cause blockade of motor function and have the potential to produce cardiac toxicity, including prolonged QTc intervals. Levobupivacaine has less cardiac toxicity than the racemic bupivacaine. Both levobupivacaine and ropivacaine produce reduced motor blockade relative to bupivacaine.[324]

**Clonidine.** Clonidine, like morphine and ziconotide, is registered with the FDA to treat severe pain. Clonidine is an alpha-2 adrenergic antagonist. It is mainly used as an adjuvant analgesic with morphine and local anesthetics. Clonidine reduces the concentration of local anesthetic required for analgesia and increases the duration of sensory block. It also increases the motor block caused by local anesthetics.[325] Because clonidine is lipophilic (as lipophilic as

### Table 11. Recommended Starting Doses of Intrathecal Medication[320]

| Drug | Recommended Intrathecal Bolus Dose |
|---|---|
| Morphine | 0.1-0.5 mg/day |
| Hydromorphone | 0.02-0.5 mg/day |
| Ziconotide | 0.5-2.4 mcg/day |
| Fentanyl | 25-75 mcg/day |
| Bupivacaine | 1-4 mg/day |
| Clonidine | 40-100 mcg/day |
| Sufentanil | 10-20 mcg/day |

*From Polyanalgesic Consensus Conference--2012: recommendations on trialing for intrathecal (intraspinal) drug delivery: report of an interdisciplinary expert panel, by Deer TR, Prager J, Levy R, et al., Neuromodulation : journal of the International Neuromodulation Society. 2012;15(5):420-435. (c) John Wiley & Sons. Reproduced with permission.*

fentanyl), it is redistributed systemically, which can lead to sedation.[326] It does not increase morphine respiratory depression but can cause hypotension, sedation, and bradycardia.[327]

**Ziconotide.** Ziconotide is a 25-amino acid derivative of an omega conotoxin derived from the venom of the conus magnus snail. It is an N-type calcium channel blocker. N-type calcium channels are found on dorsal horn presynaptic terminals. Blocking these calcium channels impairs sensory nerve transmission. Intrathecal ziconotide alone can reduce pain. There is analgesic synergy when combined with intrathecal morphine (see **Table 12**). Unfortunately ziconotide has a narrow therapeutic index and most individuals (90%) develop side effects. Ziconotide as a single agent does not cause respiratory depression. It is associated with dizziness, nausea, and asthenia. Ziconotide also is associated with psychiatric symptoms such as confusion; memory impairment; speech disorders; hallucinations; and rarely paranoia, hostility, delirium, and aphasia. The discontinuation of ziconotide reverses these side effects.[329]

### Table 12. Polyanalgesia Algorithm for Intrathecal Therapies for Cancer Pain[328]

| | |
|---|---|
| **First line** | Single-agent morphine or hydromorphone or ziconotide |
| **Second line** | Single-agent fentanyl or morphine/hydromorphone plus ziconotide or morphine/hydromorphone plus bupivacaine/clonidine |
| **Third line** | Single-agent clonidine or morphine/hydromorphone/fentanyl/bupivacaine plus clonidine ± ziconotide |

## Clinical Situation

### Robert

Robert is a 56-year-old African-American man with severe chronic obstructive pulmonary disease, coronary artery disease, and lung cancer. His cancer was discovered last year. The cancer stage was IIIA (involving mediastinal lymph nodes but potentially surgically resectable). He is undergoing chemotherapy in an attempt to reduce the size of the cancer to facilitate surgical resection. He is currently on oxycodone extended release, 10 mg every 12 hours, and occasionally takes a 5 mg oxycodone immediate-release tablet for breakthrough pain for his chest pain.

He is admitted to the hospital with new onset back pain (10 on a 10-point scale) located in the L2 region and dyspnea. He is found to have metastases in lungs, pleural effusions, and multiple vertebral metastases despite chemotherapy. He is given 4 mg IV morphine in the emergency department with moderate benefit for his back pain and is admitted to the hematology/oncology service. A palliative care team is called to assist with pain management only. When you enter the room, Robert is diaphoretic, grasping the bed rails, and crying out in pain. The nurse stops you at the door and asks if she can give him another 4 mg IV push of morphine since he tolerated it in the emergency department. Upon walking in the door, you see that Robert is in agony and respond to the nurse with "yes" as you proceed with the assessment.

**?** How may emotional and spiritual concerns be affecting his pain?

**?** What are the potential causes of his pain based on the history, physical examination, and radiographs?

**?** What additional questions should you ask in regard to his pain?

**?** What else would like to know about his response to morphine?

**?** What dosing strategy should you use to control his pain?

Robert is in acute severe pain and is unlikely to tolerate many questions until his pain is better. His back pain is likely related to vertebral metastases but could be pleuritic pain from lung metastases or a pulmonary emboli or new onset pneumonia. Adrenal metastases from lung cancer are common, and so you should do a quick PQRST assessment and review the computed tomography (CT) scan preferably with the radiologist. It would be important to know if he tolerated the morphine, if it reduced his pain, and, if so, for how long. This may give a sense of his opioid needs. Because his pain is severe and acute, a rapid dose titration strategy is in order with frequent small doses of morphine (1 mg every 1 to 5 minutes IV or SC) until his pain is significantly better. The around-the-clock dose can be estimated based on the effective dose. If the effective titrated dose that reduced his pain from a 10 to a 6 by NRS was 12 mg, then the hourly dose would be 3 mg to 4 mg per hour by PCA with a rescue dose of 2 mg to 4 mg hourly or 1 mg every 15 minutes. Careful bedside titration is safe. It is prudent to have naloxone available. You will also need to consider the oxycodone he has taken in the past 24 hours. His PCA continuous dose will need to be adjusted. He should be watched closely. It often is prudent to have the patient observed hourly. Demoralization, anxiety, depression, and catastrophizing reduces pain thresholds and opioid responses. It would be important that a chaplain, social worker, and/or psychologist see him and family. Judicial uses of opioids may allow him to participate in nonpharmacologic therapies for his "total pain." Finally, if history reveals that he is an active smoker, it would be important to anticipate nicotine withdrawal, which might hinder pain management. A nicotine patch may be helpful.

When the pain is controlled, his oncologist should be contacted and brought up to date with what has happened if he or she is unaware.

## The Case Continues

After a titrated dose of 12 mg IV morphine, a PCA is started using 4 mg per hour continuous infusion and 2 mg every hour as needed. Robert reports that his pain improves from a 10 on a 10-point scale to a 6, but the effect only lasts about 30 minutes. He has just started an infusion of morphine at 4 mg per hour. He is not exhibiting any somnolence or altered mentation. He describes radiating pain down his left leg and inability to urinate for the past 24 hours. He can stand but has some weakness on extending his left leg (4/5) with some hypersensitivity to touch in the area of pain. He has been constipated for 2 days.

**?** How should the resurgence of pain be handled?

**?** What additional tests would you want to get?

**?** What additional physical findings do you want to look for?

**?** What additional medications should be added?

Robert has just been started on a continuous infusion of morphine at 4 mg per hour and his continuous dose is not at steady state. Therefore, the as-needed dose should be adjusted 50% and he should be reassessed hourly. His continuous doses should remain the same for the next 20 to 24 hours. Be aware of the bolus effect with rescue doses. Transient nausea and other effects may be seen. If this occurs, the rescue dose could be given more frequently by the PCA at lower doses.

Robert has neuropathic radiating pain but also left leg weakness such that a spinal cord compression should be investigated with an MRI. It may be difficult for patients with back pain to stay in position for an MRI. Using a bolus of morphine before the procedure may help. For those unable to tolerate an MRI, conscious sedation may be needed or, alternatively, a CT myelogram. His constipation is likely opioid induced. However, a rectal examination for sphincter tone and perirectal sensation would be important, along with making sure he does not have a fecal impaction. His neuropathic pain could be treated with an adjuvant like gabapentin; however, in light of the potential for spinal cord compression, corticosteroids would be more appropriate.

Dexamethasone is frequently used at intervals of 6 hours. However, dexamethasone has a long half-life and can be given less frequently. Doses as high as 100 mg have been used, but most use 10 mg to 20 mg per day. The evidence for dose response is very poor. If spinal cord compression is suspected and the patient has ambulatory capacity, a spine surgeon (either orthopedic or neurosurgeon) should be consulted after informing the patient of the situation and establishing the goals of care.

*Continued on page 60*

## Opioid Titration

*Starting Dosage*

The appropriate starting dosage of an opioid depends on several factors, including the frequency and severity of pain, previous experience with opioid analgesics, recent exposure to opioids, age and body weight (especially for young children and frail older adults), and medical status. When initiating therapy for opioid-naive adults with chronic pain, the safest approach is to start with a low dosage of a short-acting oral formulation such as 5 mg of hydrocodone (in a hydrocodone/acetaminophen combination product), 2.5 mg to 5 mg of oxycodone (in an oxycodone/acetaminophen combination product), 1 mg to 2 mg of hydromorphone, or 5 mg to 10 mg of morphine every 3 to 4 hours.

As an alternative, opioid-naive adults with moderate chronic pain can be started on a modified-release formulation at a very low dose. Sustained-release morphine at a dose of 15 mg twice daily or 20 mg to 30 mg once daily is one example. However, if rapid dose titration is needed, long-acting opioids should not be used. If titration is performed with a short-acting drug, a switch to a modified-release product is done when the dose begins to stabilize. Transdermal fentanyl should be used after titration and stabilization on parenteral fentanyl.

*Dosage Escalation*

The initial opioid dosage should be titrated upward until relief is achieved or side effects supervene. A supplemental rescue dose can be offered as needed even if the baseline dose is administered as a short-acting formulation. To titrate an opioid, the dose usually is increased by 25% to 50% each increment and sometimes higher (as much as 100%) if pain is severe and the patient is medically stable. Alternatively, the dose can be increased by an amount equal to the average daily consumption of rescue doses for breakthrough pain during the previous few days.

Ideally the interval between dose escalations should be long enough to allow steady state to be approached. This is 2 to 3 days for modified-release oral formulations and 3 to 6 days for the transdermal patch. This interval usually is 5 to 7 days for methadone because of its long elimination half-life, but it can be much longer.

When pain is severe, however, more rapid dose escalation is needed. Severe pain may be treated with intravenous bolus injections at short intervals to eliminate the absorption delay that occurs after each dose. Although aggressive dosing achieves analgesic blood levels quickly, it carries the risk of delayed toxicity as levels continue to rise toward steady state after the dose stabilizes at a level that provides prompt relief. To avoid toxicity related to this "over-shooting," monitoring is needed after rapid dose adjustments until steady state is approached. If delayed somnolence or other adverse effects occur, the dose should be adjusted downward.

The dose of a short-acting drug given for breakthrough pain also must be adjusted over time to maintain effects. As noted, clinical experience suggests that the dose should remain in the range of 10% to 15% of the total oral daily dose. Exceptions are the rapid-onset fentanyl formulations, which have effects at doses that may not be proportional to the fixed schedule dose.[281] As noted earlier, it is prudent to begin treatment with rapid-onset drugs at one of the lowest available doses and then titrate based on clinical response.

There is no maximal or optimal dose of the pure mu-agonist drugs. The general rule is that doses should be titrated upward until acceptable analgesia occurs or intolerable side effects demonstrate poor responsiveness to the drug for acute pain. Most patients require a daily oral morphine equivalent of 200 mg or less. As the dose is increased, particularly to relatively high levels, toxicities, drug-related behaviors, and the burdens associated with the number of tablets or patches should be carefully reassessed.

The dosing strategy for chronic pain is distinctly different than for acute pain. Other approaches should be used rather than opioid titration and high-dose opioid therapy. Improved daily activities and physical function are better goals of therapy and more appropriate than reduced pain intensity. The utility of opioids is lower for chronic pain than for acute pain, and utility diminishes with opioid dose due to increased side effects.

Patients who develop treatment-limiting opioid side effects during dose titration are considered poorly responsive. Clinical characteristics of poor responsiveness include age (younger than 60 years), neuropathic pain, depression, anxiety, and incident pain.[330] In these cases, another therapeutic strategy must be selected (**Table 13**). Opioid rotation is the most common approach in this setting.[262]

## Table 13. Clinical Strategies to Address Poor Opioid Responsiveness[170]

| Approach | Options |
| --- | --- |
| Identify a more effective opioid | Opioid rotation |
| Open the "therapeutic window" | More aggressive side effect management |
| Add a systemic or spinal coanalgesic to reduce the opioid requirement | Coadministered NSAID, nontraditional analgesic, or a trial of neuraxial analgesia |
| Add a nonpharmacological approach to reduce the opioid requirement | Neural blockade, a neurostimulatory approach, or psychological or rehabilitative therapy |

*Reprinted from* The Lancet, *377(9784), RK Portenoy, Treatment of Cancer Pain, 2236-2247, ©2011, with permission from Elsevier.*

# Opioid Rotation

When patients experience intolerable side effects or persistent pain despite escalating dosages of opioids, physicians may consider switching to a different opioid medication. Using a conversion table, a physician can compare potencies across different modes of administration (eg, oral versus IV) and different types of opioids (see Table 7). These values provide a guide that helps clinicians select a safe and effective dose of the new drug. It is important to recognize that the equianalgesic doses stated on conversion tables are based on older, single-dose studies and that subsequent studies have revealed wide variability in conversion ratios.[331] Consequently, the equianalgesic dose table should only be used as a general guide.

Newer guidelines for opioid rotation emphasize safety by incorporating a two-step process to select the starting dose of the new drug (**Table 14**).[263] The first step involves calculating the equianalgesic dose (Table 7), then reducing the calculated dose to account for incomplete

## Table 14. Guidelines for Opioid Rotation

**Step 1**

- Select the new drug based on prior experience, availability, cost, and other factors.
- Calculate the equianalgesic dose from the equianalgesic dose table (see Table 7).
- If switching to an opioid other than methadone or fentanyl, identify an automatic dose reduction window of 25%-50% less than the calculated equianalgesic dose.
- If switching to methadone, the automatic dose reduction window is 75%-90%; rarely convert to methadone at a dose higher than 100 mg/day.
- If switching to transdermal fentanyl, do not use an automatic dose reduction; use the calculated equianalgesic dose included in the package insert.
- Select a dose closer to the lower bound (25% reduction) or the upper bound (50% reduction) of the automatic dose reduction window on the basis of a judgment that the equianalgesic dose table is relatively more or less applicable to the characteristics of the regimen or patient:
  » Select a dose closer to the upper bound if the patient is receiving a relatively high dose of the current opioid, is not Caucasian, or is elderly or medically frail.
  » Select a dose closer to the lower bound if upper-bound criteria are not met and if being switched to a different route using the same drug.

**Step 2**

- Based on assessment of pain severity and other medical or psychosocial characteristics, increase or decrease the calculated dose by 15%-30% to enhance the likelihood the initial dose will be effective or, conversely, is unlikely to cause withdrawal or side effects.
- Assess response and titrate the dose of the new opioid regimen to optimize outcomes.
- If a supplemental dose is used as needed, calculate this dose at 5%-15% of the total daily opioid dose and administer at an appropriate interval; transmucosal fentanyl formulations are exceptions and always should be initiated at one of the lower doses.

*Reprinted from The Lancet, 377(9784), RK Portenoy, Treatment of Cancer Pain, 2236-2247, ©2011, with permission from Elsevier.*

cross-tolerance and individual variation. The second step involves additional dose adjustment based on clinical factors. For example, a patient who is experiencing poor pain control and mental clouding while taking long-acting oxycodone at a dose of 60 mg twice daily might be considered for a switch to an alternative drug. There are no data to inform the selection of this drug, and the decision usually is based on availability, cost, convenience, and previous experience. If morphine is selected, the 120 mg daily dosage of oxycodone is roughly equianalgesic to a 180 mg daily dosage of morphine. If a reduction of 25% is applied, the daily dosage of morphine would be 135 mg. If the patient is medically frail, this might be decreased a small amount (to 120 mg/day), and a long-acting morphine then might be started at a dose of 60 mg twice daily. A rescue dose also can be offered, such as short-acting morphine, 15 mg every 2 hours as needed.

The method of opioid rotation shown in Table 14 can also be applied to drugs that are administered by other routes. It is prudent to reduce the calculated equianalgesic dose even if the same drug is to be administered by a different route given interindividual variation in bioavailability that characterizes this class.

## Clinical Situation

### Robert's Case Continues (continued from page 57)

After receiving 4 mg per hour of intravenous morphine over the past hour and a dose of 10 mg intravenous dexamethasone, Robert relaxes and reports his pain at a 5 out of 10. Based on his opioid use, you start morphine via PCA and schedule his intravenous steroids. Robert receives an MRI scan, which shows metastases at the second and third lumbar vertebrae with extension into the epidural space. The hematology/oncology team consults with neurosurgery and radiation oncology clinicians. The next day, Robert reports that his pain is about 4 out of 10 and is much improved. He has used 96 mg intravenous morphine in the past 24 hours. His neurological status has improved and is back to baseline after the steroids were initiated. Because of his poor performance status and comorbidities, the specialists feel that he is a high-risk surgical candidate, and the patient opts for palliative radiation only. The nurse calls you because Robert is starting to have severe myoclonus. It is interfering with his ability to sleep and eat.

 What are the best options for managing opioid-induced myoclonus?

Common side effects of opioids include constipation, myoclonus, nausea, somnolence, dry mouth, and pruritus. If bothersome to the patient, myoclonus can be addressed in a number of ways. If the symptoms are distressing to the patient, a trial of opioid dose reduction, rotation, or the addition of a benzodiazepine may be helpful. Adding a benzodiazepine, however, increases the risk for cognitive impairment, falls, respiratory depression, and sleep-disordered breathing, which is common with chronic obstructive pulmonary disease (COPD). Therefore, benzodiazepines should not be used in this case. Gabapentin has been reported anecdotally to help with myoclonus and may allow for an opioid dose reduction. Gabapentin can cause sedation and so should be titrated slowly. Finally, some people tolerate myoclonus of a mild nature that does not impair their function. A final alternative is a "wait and see" approach. Physicians often fail to systematically assess patients for opioid toxicity. In one study, patients on opioids had 10 related symptoms while those in pain and not on opioids had three. It would be prudent to ask Robert about nightmares, vivid dreams, and visual hallucinations.

### The Case Concludes

Robert's myoclonus resolves when the morphine is rotated to a hydromorphone PCA. He is tolerating palliative radiation and some limited physical therapy. A few days prior to discharge, you recommend a transition to oral pain medication. Robert is discharged on morphine extended release 100 mg every 8 hours based on his PCA requirements, with 30 mg of immediate-release morphine every 4 hours as needed for breakthrough pain and a tapering dexamethasone dose after radiation. He has a follow-up appointment in the palliative care clinic and hematology/oncology clinic.

## Managing Opioid Side Effects

Effective treatment of side effects increases the likelihood of a favorable response to opioids and is consistent with the broader goals of palliative care. Common adverse effects include constipation and GI-related symptoms (eg, nausea, vomiting, anorexia, bloating, early satiety) as well as somnolence, immunosuppression, mental clouding, falls, and confusion. There are many other potential side effects. Most clinicians appreciate the possibility of dry mouth, urinary retention, or myoclonus. Less well-known are the effects of hypogonadism (eg, fatigue, depressed mood, sexual dysfunction, loss of muscle mass) and sleep-disordered breathing. Concern also exists about respiratory depressant effects. Side effects are both dosage related and idiosyncratic; in the context of serious illness, many adverse effects are determined by more than one factor. Whenever a side effect interferes with therapy, an assessment is needed to establish its etiologies and develop a responsive plan of care.

### Cardiovascular Adverse Effects

Opioid therapy is associated with increased cardiovascular deaths on par with NSAIDs.[332] Patients on long-term opioids can develop myocardial infarction and heart failure as a result of opioid therapy. There is a 77% increased risk regardless of the opioid.[333,334] A large cohort study has confirmed the increased risk of myocardial infarction and the need for revascularization for patients on long-term opioids.[335] Opioids reduce testosterone levels and increase the incidence of metabolic syndrome and insulin resistance.[336,337] Given these risks, depending on life expectancy and goals of care, consideration should be given to screening for a lipid disorder and treatment with low-dose aspirin or statins. One study found that testosterone replacement in those with opioid-induced hypogonadism did not improve leptin levels, C-reactive protein levels, insulin sensitivity, glucose levels, oral glucose tolerance tests, or hyperlipidemia.[338]

## Arrhythmia and QTc prolongation

Three opioids are associated with prolonged QTc intervals in electrocardiogram, but only one, methadone, is associated with torsades de pointes. Oxycodone in high doses interferes with repolarization by blocking potassium repolarizing channels. Oxycodone doses of 100 mg or greater increase QTc intervals by 10 milliseconds on average (95% CI, 2-19), whereas neither morphine nor tramadol were noted to increase the QTc interval.[339] No incidence of torsades de pointes has been reported with oxycodone.[340] Buprenorphine is 75- to 100-fold less potent than methadone in blocking the expression of the potassium channel protein needed for cardiac repolarization (human ether-a-go-go [hERG]) and is 3.5-fold less potent than fentanyl.[341] Increased QTc intervals were noted in US studies of transdermal buprenorphine.[342] Multiple studies using large doses of sublingual buprenorphine as maintenance therapy have not demonstrated a prolonged QTc interval with buprenorphine or demonstrated a resolution of a prolonged QTc interval when buprenorphine was substituted for methadone.[342-345] There is much experience with transdermal buprenorphine in Europe, with doses of 35, 52, and 70 mcg per hour without reported arrhythmia or QTc prolongation.[346-349] There have been no reports of increased arrhythmias with buprenorphine and no recommendation for electrocardiogram monitoring for QTc prolongation.[340] Fentanyl actually has a protective effect on anesthetic-induced QTc prolongation. There are no concerns about fentanyl causing prolongation.[350,351]

Methadone has been associated with QTc prolongation and torsades de pointes. Mortality from torsades de pointes is as high as 17%.[352] Methadone (R) enantiomer, the enantiomer that binds the opioid receptor and is responsible for analgesia, also is responsible for the QTc prolongation.[353] The (R) enantiomer blocks hERG, which is critical for cardiac repolarization.[341] The risk of torsades de pointes is particularly high when the QTc is greater than 500 milliseconds or if there is a greater than 60-millisecond increase in QTc interval from baseline.[354,355] There is an increased risk for torsades de pointes if there is hypokalemia, hypomagnesemia, cardiovascular disease, silent prolonged QTc interval, family history of sudden death, and polypharmacy, which may include medications that also prolong the QTc interval (haloperidol, tricyclic antidepressant, chlorpromazine).[356] Medications that block CYP3A4/5 and CYP2B6 (eg, fluconazole, erythromycin, clarithromycin, ciprofloxacin, fluoxetine) will increase the risk for torsades de pointes by delaying (R)-methadone clearance.[356] Recent recommendations have been published regarding monitoring individuals who are taking methadone.[279] Individuals receiving disease-modifying therapy and cancer survivors should undergo electrocardiogram monitoring as recommended by the American Pain Society. Monitoring QTc intervals may not be appropriate for hospice patients with a primary goal of comfort and very limited life expectancy.

## Xerostomia

The occurrence of xerostomia for patients receiving opioids ranges between 33% and 70%. For those with advanced cancer, the prevalence of xerostomia is as high as 95%.[357] Individuals taking long-term opioids for noncancer pain have a 50% risk of experiencing xerostomia.[358] Xerostomia also occurs as a result of radiation therapy to the head and neck region, chemotherapy, or use of drugs that have anticholinergic activity. Tolerance does not develop to xerostomia. Treatment recommendations are largely based on expert opinion. Saliva substitution and pilocarpine have been reported to be helpful.[359,360]

## Opioid-Induced Urinary Dysfunction

Urinary retention related to opioids occurs in 3.8% to 18.1% of patients receiving opioids for postoperative pain.[361,362] Urinary retention occurs more commonly with spinal than parenteral opioids.[363] Opioids reduce detrusor muscle tone and force of contraction as well as the sensation of bladder fullness and urge to void. The result is an inhibition of the voiding reflex. Opioids do not alter urinary sphincter tone.[364] The adverse effects on bladder function are reversed by naloxone. These adverse effects are in part due to peripheral mu receptor activation, which can be blocked by methylnaltrexone without reversing analgesia.[365] There is no evidence that opioid rotation improves urinary retention.

## Constipation

Opioid-induced constipation (OIC) is common and presumably worsened by advanced age, immobility, poor diet, intraabdominal pathology, neuropathy, hypercalcemia, or the use of other constipating drugs.[366,367] Contributing causes should be minimized, if possible, and symptomatic therapies should be pursued. Prophylactic treatment to prevent constipation at the time an opioid is prescribed is appropriate for patients with predisposing factors, which is common in populations with serious or life-threatening illnesses.

Opioids produce constipation by inhibiting longitudinal smooth muscle, thus reducing peristalsis, increasing contraction of circular muscle resulting in segmentation, increasing absorption of fluid from the bowel, and impairing secretions. In addition, opioids impair sphincter function.[367,368] The opioid receptors on smooth muscle and enteric neurons within the submucosal and myenteric plexus are largely responsible for OIC.[368] The clinical presentation of OIC does not differ from that of functional constipation except that the constipation occurs with opioid treatment. OIC is identified on the basis of the Rome III criteria definition of constipation.[369] The most common symptoms used as inclusion criteria in these trials are fewer than three bowel movements per week, straining, hard stools, and sensation of incomplete evacuation. OIC can occur even at low dosages of opioids[370] and can occur at any time after initiation of opioid therapy.[371] Nausea, vomiting, and gastroesophageal reflux are the other symptoms associated with OIC.[372] All opioids can cause constipation, and this can occur when the drug is given by any route of administration. Considering the influence of receptors in the gut, it is likely that oral administration is more likely to produce constipation than other drug delivery routes. The observation that transdermal fentanyl causes less constipation than oral morphine supports this conclusion.[291]

Dietary changes (eg, more fruits, high-fiber foods, hydration) may be appropriate for some patients with OIC, but the strength of evidence for benefit is low. Fiber supplements should be avoided. During treatment, attention must be paid to privacy; a private commode with easy access is essential. Expense is another concern because the high cost of some laxatives can interfere with compliance.

**Treatment for Constipation**

Few studies help define the comparative effectiveness of various constipation strategies and the potential value of dose escalation or combination therapy. Treatment usually begins with a simple oral regimen using an osmotic agent (eg, a poorly absorbed sugar such as lactulose, sorbitol, or polyethylene glycol) followed by a stimulant laxative (eg, senna or bisacodyl). Dosages may be increased, and the various agents may be administered in combination, as needed. **Table 15** provides an example of a laxative regimen.

## Table 15. An Effective Stepwise Laxative Regimen

| Step | Medication | Regimen |
|------|-----------|---------|
| 1 | Polyethylene glycol, sorbitol, or lactulose | 17 g polyethylene glycol in 6 oz of water; 30 mL of sorbitol or lactulose |
| 2 | Add senna | 2 tabs daily |
| 3 | Increase senna | 2 tabs twice daily |
| 4 | Increase senna *and add* | 4 tabs twice daily |
| | sorbitol *or* | 30 mL twice daily |
| | polyethylene glycol *or* | 17 g in 8 oz of water daily |
| | bisacodyl | 2 tabs twice daily |
| 5 | Increase sorbitol *or* | 30 mL three times daily |
| | polyethylene glycol *or* | 17 g in 8 oz of water twice daily |
| | bisacodyl | 3 tabs three times daily |

taking chronic opioids have low bone mass. There is a direct relationship between reduced free testosterone and a low bone mineral density ($P = .02$).[406] Individuals taking morphine dosages greater than 100 mg per day or an equivalent are at particular risk and should have bone mineral density and free testosterone levels measured if they have been on opioids for a long period of time, if consistent with goals of care and life expectancy.[407] Alternatively, one could consider preventive bisphosphonate therapy for patients at risk for osteoporosis or with preexisting osteoporosis who will remain on long-term opioid therapy.

## Opioid-Induced Endocrinopathies

Opioids influence every hormone released from the anterior pituitary. Gonadotropins are particularly adversely affected. The prevalence of symptoms and/or chemical evidence of hypogonadism is 75% to 100% with patients on long-term opioids.[408] Opioids inhibit gonadotropin-releasing hormones and thus cause hypogonadotropic hypogonadism. Opioids also impair the hypothalamic-pituitary-adrenal axis, which results in reductions of dehydroepiandrosterone (DHEA) and conjugated DHEA (DHEAS).[336,337] Reduced testosterone is associated with metabolic syndrome, insulin resistance, fatigue, mood changes, impotence, and loss of libido. Long-term testosterone deficiency is associated with sarcopenia and osteoporosis. Reduced pulsatile release of gonadotropins in women leads to oligomenorrhea or amenorrhea, infertility, sexual dysfunction, estrogen deficiency, hot flashes, and fatigue. Prolactin levels are increased, which causes galactorrhea.[336]

Both estrogen and testosterone deficiency in women lead to osteoporosis.[409-411] Opioid-induced endocrinopathies occur with oral, parenteral, transdermal, and spinal opioids. Rotating routes of administration does not appear to reduce the risk.[412] Both testosterone and cortisol levels are reduced within 1 to 4 hours after a single administration of opioid, and they return to normal levels within 24 hours.[410,413,414]

Chronic opioids and, in particular, the use of long-acting opioids reduce free and total testosterone.[415] Not all men receiving long-term opioid therapy will develop hypogonadism.[416-419] Sexual dysfunction may only be partly related to the reduction of testosterone. Sexual function may also be reduced with opioids and normal testosterone levels, which will not respond to testosterone replacement.[420,421] Testosterone replacement for opioid-induced testosterone deficiency is not FDA-approved. However, studies demonstrate improvement in sexual function, mood, hot flashes, fatigue, and well-being. Benefits are generally partial, and symptoms do not fully resolve.[409,422] Testosterone is necessary for endogenous opioid activity and is important to binding opioid ligands to receptors. Testosterone also modulates dopamine and norepinephrine activity. As a result, low levels of testosterone can lower pain thresholds and increase pain sensitivity. This may lead to poor pain control as well as sleep disturbances.[411] Quantitative sensory studies have shown that testosterone replacement improves pressure pain thresholds, mechanical pain thresholds, and cold pressor pain but does not appear to improve self-reported pain.[423] Low testosterone levels predispose individuals to inflammation, poor tissue healing, and compression fractures,[411,424-426] which can lead to chronic pain.

Women receiving long-term opioid therapy have an increased risk of bone fractures directly related to reduced estrogen and testosterone.[39,427] Little is known about the benefits of estrogen and/or testosterone replacement in reducing falls and fractures for women on chronic opioid therapy.

Adrenal androgens are reduced in men and women receiving long-term opioid therapy.[410,428-430] Opioids cause a reduction in DHEA, which is a sensitive marker of adrenal insufficiency. Adrenocorticotropic hormone levels are in the normal range. Low levels of DHEA and hypoadrenalism result in additional sexual dysfunction and fatigue for both men and women.[409,428,429] DHEA levels are below normal in 67% of people taking opioids compared with 6% of those who are opioid naïve. Methadone produces a progressive decrease in cortisol blood levels that is dose dependent. Fentanyl has greater adverse effects on corticosteroid levels than morphine.[431,432]

Tests for opioid-induced endocrinopathies should not be routine but based upon signs and symptoms of deficiencies of androgen, estrogen, or corticosteroid. Sex hormone binding globulin, luteinizing hormone, follicle-stimulating hormone, total and free testosterone, DHEAS, and DHEA should be evaluated. Based upon signs and symptoms, physicians may need to perform specific tests for adrenal function.[337] Tests should be done in the morning, the time when testosterone is at the highest plasma level.[433] For women, estradiol levels, DHEA, DHEAS, and testosterone levels as well as bone density studies may guide therapy.[429] Replacement testosterone doses for women are approximately one-quarter to one-third of doses used for men.

Management includes tapering opioids if possible and discontinuing opioid therapy. This is more likely to be successful for cancer survivors. There are weak data that rotation to buprenorphine or tapentadol may have less adverse effects on hypothalamic function.[419,434] The target testosterone level for men is between 400 ng/dL and 700 ng/dL and for women, 20 ng/dL to 80 ng/dL. Individuals on testosterone replacement therapy should have testosterone levels, calcium, lipid profiles, coagulation studies, hepatic function, and a complete blood count drawn periodically.[433,435] Testosterone replacement therapy does have risks. Replacement may worsen sleep-disordered breathing and hyperlipidemia and may cause hypercalcemia and polycythemia.[411,436]

### Opioid-Induced Immunosuppression

Morphine suppresses cellular immunity and decreases resistance to bacterial infections.[437-439] Over a century ago, guinea pigs treated with morphine were shown to be at an increased risk of developing pneumonia.[412] Endogenous opioids are not immunosuppressive. The immunosuppressive effects of exogenous opioids appear to be mediated by peripheral and central mu receptors. There is a bidirectional relationship between opioids and peripheral immunocytes. Peripheral immunocytes release endogenous opioids, which facilitates analgesia. Immunocytes also express mu receptors, which enable opioids to feed back and modulate immune function.[440,441] Morphine decreases the effectiveness of natural and acquired immunity, interfering with important intracellular pathways involved in immune regulation. Not all opioids induce the same immunosuppressive effects. For example, fentanyl is more immunosuppressive than buprenorphine. The impact of the opioid-mediated immune effects may be particularly problematic in selective vulnerable populations, such as older or immunocompromised patients.[437]

## Somnolence

Opioids are thought to induce sedation via anticholinergic effects.[442] Some patients initially are sleepy because sleep deprivation associated with pain is finally relieved. Some patients, however, experience long-lasting somnolence, mental clouding, or confusion, and some experience other effects on higher cortical functioning such as mood disturbance (typically dysphoria) or perceptual disturbances. Frank delirium, in which any or all of these effects are combined with a fluctuating level of consciousness, may be caused or worsened by opioids and is common in the setting of far-advanced illness. If somnolence or mental clouding occurs when opioid therapy has begun or when the dose is increased, this may signal poor opioid responsiveness and indicate the need for an alternative approach, such as opioid rotation or reducing other psychotropic medications.

In some animal studies, tolerance to opioid-induced sedation occurs more quickly than tolerance to respiratory depression.[443] Sedation is particularly prevalent with initiation of opioid therapy or with rapid titration. Psychostimulants improve subjective sedation and psychomotor performance impaired by opioids.[444] The usual dosage of methylphenidate is 10 mg to 15 mg per day, which improves opioid-induced drowsiness compared with placebo.[445,446] A side benefit to methylphenidate in these studies was reduced pain, which allowed for reduction in opioid dosages. Other therapies that anecdotally are helpful are donepezil, dextroamphetamine, and modafinil.[447]

## Mood Disorders

Opioids were commonly used for depression before effective antidepressants became available. Opioids were abandoned after the introduction of antidepressants because of the risk of addiction.[448] Low-dose buprenorphine has been effective in reducing suicidal ideation for depressed individuals without altering depression.[449] Buprenorphine appears to reduce affective symptoms (painful feelings of rejection or abandonment) that precipitate suicidal ideation without influencing neurovegetative symptoms and reduced sense of pleasure.[449]

High-dose opioids are associated with depressed mood in individuals without depression prior to opioid therapy.[7,8,32] Individuals who become depressed on opioids may have improved mood (and perhaps better pain control) with reduction in opioid doses or tapering opioids completely. It is not known if antidepressants ameliorate opioid-induced depression.

## Myoclonus

The incidence of myoclonus on opioids is 3% to 87% depending on the opioid dose, duration of opioid therapy, and the presence of certain opioid metabolites. It is often observed when the patient becomes drowsy or just before entering light sleep.[450,451] Myoclonus is generally mild and self-limiting but can cause clinical distress in a subset of patients. Myoclonus can reduce physical function and worsen pain through involuntary movements. Myoclonus is not reversible by naloxone. Patients and families need reassurance; treatment may or may not be necessary. If the involuntary movements are distressing, opioid rotation[452] or a trial of a benzodiazepine may be helpful, but one should be careful about combining opioids with benzodiazepines because of additive risks and side effects. Patients with symptomatic myoclonus often complain of difficulties feeding themselves, holding a cup of coffee, or falling asleep because of involuntary jerking. Medications reported to help treat myoclonus include baclofen, dantrolene, haloperidol, and anticonvulsants such as gabapentin and valproate.[64,412,450,453-456] Paradoxically, gabapentin can also cause myoclonus when used as an adjuvant analgesic.[457-459]

## Opioid-Induced Delirium

The pathophysiology of opioid-induced delirium is in part related to the anticholinergic effects of opioids.[460] Individuals receiving parenteral morphine doses of 90 mg per day or greater have a 1.7-times higher risk for delirium. Individuals with cancer who are taking opioids have a 40% greater risk of developing delirium than those who are not taking opioids.[461] In a study that involved 114 patients who were started on morphine, oxycodone, or fentanyl, the incidence of delirium was 28.9% in the morphine group, 19.5% in the oxycodone group, and 8.6% in the fentanyl group. There was a significant difference between the morphine and fentanyl groups (Fisher's exact test, $P = .04$) but not between the morphine and oxycodone groups nor between the oxycodone and fentanyl groups.[462]

Tramadol is a strong risk factor for postoperative delirium and has been reported to produce both acute and chronic delirium in various settings.[463] Individuals at risk include those with renal dysfunction, active infections, metabolic abnormalities, prior cognitive impairment, dehydration, or multiple psychotropic medications. Management includes reducing psychotropics, screening and treating other reversible causes of delirium, reducing opioid dosages by 25%, or rotating opioids. Hydration may reduce delirium. Naloxone does not reverse opioid-induced delirium. Antipsychotics have been recommended for patients who are terminally ill and imminently dying; however, there are no randomized trials that have demonstrated benefits to the use of any antipsychotics for opioid-induced delirium.[358] Anecdotally, donepezil has been shown to improve opioid-induced delirium.[464]

## Sleep-Disordered Breathing

Long-term opioid use is associated with sleep-disordered breathing, which includes central sleep apnea and ataxic breathing and can lead to hypoxemia and carbon dioxide retention.[465] Seventy-five percent of patients taking opioids for 6 months will have sleep-disordered breathing, while in the general population this is seen in only 3% to 20% of people.[466] Ten percent of individuals on stable dosages of methadone will have some degree of hypoxemia, defined as an oxyhemoglobin saturation of less than 90%.[467] The adverse effects of opioids on breathing are dose dependent. Sleep-disordered breathing (defined as an apnea hypopnea index greater than 5) occurs in 92% of patients on 200 mg of morphine or equivalents per day. Sixty percent of patients taking less than 200 mg of morphine or its equivalents per day will have sleep-disordered breathing; in the general population prevalence is 5%.[468] Sleep-disordered breathing occurs during rapid eye movement (REM) sleep, and oxygen desaturation usually occurs during non-REM sleep. Opioids reduce the respiratory rate with compensated tidal volume at low dosages. This maintains minute ventilation. At high dosages, opioids will reduce both respiratory rate and tidal volume, leading to reduced minute ventilation, hypoxia, and hypercapnea.[469]

The respiratory rate is governed by two interconnecting pacemaker centers within the medulla. The more rostral pre-Botzinger complex contains neurons with mu receptors. These particular neurons act as pacemakers to initiate inspiration. The more caudal retro-trapezoid nucleus/parafacial respiratory group contains a pacemaker that, when activated, inhibits the more rostral complex to initiate expiration. Opioids hyperpolarize the pre-Botzinger complex, which abolishes synaptic drive to inspiratory muscles. Opioids do not interfere with the oscillating interactions between the two respiratory centers. The result is a delay in inspiration and an occasional missed cycle leading to ataxic breathing and potentially apnea.[470] In animal studies, continuous morphine leads to analgesic tolerance and tolerance to sedation before tolerance develops to adverse effects on respiratory drive.[443] Patients with preexisting sleep apnea may be particularly prone to opioid-related sleep-disordered breathing. Paradoxically, those with a lower body mass index are at greater risk for opioid sleep-disordered breathing.[468]

Management includes opioid dose reduction and, if necessary for pain control, addition of an adjuvant analgesic. Rotation to another opioid may be considered, although there are no studies to validate the practice based on improved sleep-disordered breathing. This also is true for buprenorphine.[471] Caution should be exercised when prescribing benzodiazepines and benzodiazepine-like "Z-medications" (eg, zolpidem and related sedatives) because of additive risks and side effects. Continuous positive airway pressure may be helpful for patients experiencing opioid-induced sleep-disordered breathing.[472]

### Life-Threatening Respiratory Depression: Bradypnea and Hypotension

Hypotension may occur in individuals who are dehydrated when started on opioid therapy. This may be due to the sympatholytic effects of opioids. Respiratory depression (respiratory rate lower than 10 breaths per minute) is usually accompanied by sedation. Physiologic tolerance to opioid-related analgesia does not necessarily parallel tolerance to respiratory effects. Individuals on large dosages of oral morphine (more than 100 mg per day) or equivalents are at a substantial risk for overdose.[473] There is an almost nine-fold risk of respiratory depression when patients are taking more than 100 mg of morphine or equivalents per day. Approximately 12% of overdoses are fatal.

If opioid overdose is suspected and the patient is drowsy and breathing fewer than 8 to 10 times per minute or hypoxic due to hypoventilation, the opioid should be stopped and the patient monitored until the medication wears off. Verbal or gentle mechanical stimulation may be needed to maintain arousal. Subsequently the opioid usually can be restarted at a lower dose. On the rare occasion that naloxone is necessary, the best approach is to dilute naloxone to 40 mcg/mL saline and give 1 mL intravenously or subcutaneously every 1 to 5 minutes until bradypnea resolves (respiratory rate higher than 10 breaths minute). If there is no response, the dose should be increased every 2 minutes to a maximum of 15 mg. If there is no resolution in respiratory depression after the administration of 15 mg of naloxone, it is unlikely that the cause of the respiratory depression is opioid overdose.[474] The target is the "window" between reversing bradypnea and reversing analgesia, so administering small doses at frequent intervals is the best strategy.[475] Repeating the naloxone administration process or providing a naloxone infusion after initial dosing may be necessary because naloxone has a shorter half-life (30 minutes) than the opioid. This is particularly important for patients taking methadone, sustained-release opioids, or transdermal fentanyl. Naloxone can also be given intranasally if venous access or a subcutaneous line is not available.[476] Buprenorphine-induced respiratory depression is unique and requires larger doses of naloxone. In this situation, 2 mg to 4 mg of naloxone should be given as a bolus and 2 mg given parenterally over 90 minutes.[477] Opioids blunt the respiratory response to hypoxia, and opioid-treated patients who develop pneumonia or pulmonary embolism may develop sudden respiratory compromise requiring opioid dose reduction.

## Opioid Risk Management

During the past 2 decades the substantial increase in prescription drug abuse and overdose deaths in the United States[478] has paralleled an increase in the use of opioid therapy for patients with chronic noncancer pain. These phenomena have raised substantial concerns on the part of the clinical community, regulators, policy makers, and those in law enforcement, and major changes in regulations governing prescribing are being implemented as a result.[204] Although clinicians must continue to advocate strongly for ready access to opioids for legitimate medical purposes, it is essential that they also acknowledge the serious nature of drug abuse and addiction and the obligation to minimize these outcomes if possible.[479,480]

Risk assessment requires an understanding of key phenomena.[481] Addiction and physical dependence are different and should not be confused in the clinical setting; the susceptibility to a withdrawal syndrome upon sudden cessation should never be stigmatized by the label of "addiction." *Pseudoaddiction* is a poorly characterized phenomenon and is best understood as the potential for unrelieved pain to drive aberrant behavior in some people. Importantly, pseudoaddiction and addiction can coexist, and the possibility of the former should not undermine the diagnosis of addiction or the appropriate management strategies to deal with seriously problematic drug-related behavior. Drug abuse refers to the use of any drug outside of social norms, and in the medical context also refers to egregious misuse of prescription drugs. Misuse and abuse of prescription drugs also may be characterized generically as aberrant drug-related behavior or nonadherence behavior[480] (see the sidebar on page 73 for definitions of these terms).

# Definitions[482]

**Addiction**.* *Addiction* is a primary, chronic, and neurobiological disease. Its development and manifestations are influenced by genetic, psychosocial, and environmental factors. It is characterized by behaviors that include one or more of the following: impaired control over drug use, compulsive use, continued use despite harm, and craving.

**Physical dependence**.* *Physical dependence* is a state of adaptation indicated by a medication class-specific withdrawal syndrome that can be produced by abrupt cessation, rapid dosage reduction, decreasing blood level of the drug, or administration of an antagonist.

**Pseudoaddiction**. *Pseudoaddiction* is an iatrogenic syndrome with behaviors that mimic addiction and are driven by unrelieved pain. It is caused by inadequately prescribed analgesics, leading to patient demands for opioid analgesia that the care team considers excessive. When patients are provided with adequate dosages of medications at regular dosing intervals, the drug-seeking behaviors generally cease.

*From Definitions Related to the Use of Opioids for the Treatment of Pain, by the American Pain Society, 2008, American Pain Society website, www.americanpainsociety.org. © 2008 by American Pain Society. Reprinted with permission.*

All prescribers, including those in the palliative care setting, are recommended to perform universal risk management[483] during opioid therapy. Managing the risks of abuse, addiction, and diversion can reduce both individual harm and potential harm to public health. The ability to manage risk also enhances expertise in prescribing to diverse populations, including those characterized by comorbid substance use disorder.

Many physicians are reluctant to prescribe opioids because of misconceptions about their effects. Nurses may be reluctant to administer (and patients may be reluctant to use) morphine or other opioids for many of the same reasons. Similarly, patients and their family caregivers may have strong negative feelings about opioid analgesics. Healthcare professionals must be knowledgeable to avoid reinforcing fears and to dispel concerns that interfere with safe and effective prescribing. Some of these misconceptions were noted previously; the following and others are worthy of emphasis.

## Opioids and Addiction

Clinicians need to clearly understand the differences between physical dependence, pseudo-addiction, and addiction (see sidebar). Addiction, now more specifically described as opioid use disorder, is a serious biopsychosocial disease with a strong genetic basis. Some patients with serious or life-threatening illnesses will have this disease or the biological basis for it. The most accepted risk factors are a personal history of alcoholism or drug abuse, a family history of alcoholism or drug abuse, and major psychiatric disorder. The de novo development of addiction in a patient without any of these characteristics is distinctly rare. The need to prescribe opioids to patients who have a history of drug abuse or other predisposing factors to addiction is relatively common. The most prudent course for prescribers is to adopt a universal precautions risk management strategy. A small number of "at-risk" opioid-naive patients in pain who might abuse their therapeutically appropriate opioid analgesics can be identified by evaluating their past history of substance use and psychopathology. People with a history of alcohol or cocaine abuse and alcohol or drug-related convictions require more intense assessment and follow-up for evidence of misuse if opioids are prescribed. In addition, pain experienced by patients who are "at-risk" for abuse can be managed with prescriptions of small quantities of opioids and weekly prescriptions.[484] This approach ensures that all patients are appropriately assessed for risk and that actions commensurate with risk are taken to minimize the adverse outcomes of abuse, addiction, and diversion (**Table 16**). Clinicians cannot discount the importance of these latter outcomes; rather, they must recognize their characteristics, assess appropriately, and plan a management strategy to minimize risk at all times.

Patients with a past history of an addiction disorder may be fearful of reactivating their addiction behaviors and thus reluctant to embark on opioid therapy. Some see staying sober as a primary life goal and will refuse opioid therapy. Several opioid-specific screening tools are available for screening and monitoring for abuse. Many screening tools contain items on personal and family history of addiction and other risk factors such as age, sexual abuse, and psychological disease. Some tools are specific to pain management, while others assess risk factors for addiction in general.[484] These instruments help in clinical decision making but should not necessarily be viewed as diagnostic for addiction. Many of the questionnaires have not been validated, and the psychometric properties of these instruments are considered to be weak. Self-report instruments have limitations because patients may not always be truthful in their responses. Nonetheless, it is a widely accepted best practice to adopt one of the screening tools that are available and use it on a regular basis.[484] Special considerations include comanagement with an addiction specialist and providing counseling to optimize pain control and minimize psychological comorbidity.

In contrast to addiction, physical dependence is an expected result of long-term opioid treatment. It refers to the potential for withdrawal and is rarely a clinical problem as long as the dose is not abruptly lowered or an opioid antagonist administered. Opioid withdrawal is characterized by the presence of one or more of a variable group of symptoms and signs, including tremulousness, anxiety, insomnia, tachycardia, tachypnea, hypertension, nausea and vomiting, diarrhea, piloerection, and sweating. It is distinctly uncomfortable but not life-threatening unless medical comorbidities increase the risks associated with tachycardia and hypertension. In the vast majority of patients, if a treatment such as radiation therapy reduces the source of pain, an opioid can be tapered off without inducing serious withdrawal symptoms. Physical dependence should be anticipated and managed. It should never be confused with or labeled as addiction[482] or used to justify withholding treatment.

## Table 16. Principles of Risk Management During Opioid Therapy for Pain

| Principle | Goals | Strategies | Comment |
|---|---|---|---|
| Stratify risk | Clarify the likelihood of future aberrant drug-related behavior. | Consider higher risk if<br>• history of alcohol or drug abuse<br>• family history of alcohol or drug abuse<br>• major psychiatric disorder<br>Other factors that suggest risk:<br>• cancer associated with heavy alcohol use or smoking<br>• current heavy smoking<br>• younger age<br>• history of automobile accidents, chronic unemployment, limited support system<br>Factors that may mitigate risk:<br>• poor performance status<br>• limited prognosis<br>• active recovery program | All patients should undergo risk assessment and stratification.<br><br>Although many questionnaires have been developed to predict aberrant behavior or addiction, the clinical assessment is generally used in practice. |
| Structure therapy commensurate with risk | Develop practices to match monitoring with risk and, when needed, help patients maintain control. | Strategies include<br>• use of urine drug screening<br>• small amounts prescribed<br>• no use of short-acting drugs<br>• use of one pharmacy<br>• pill counts at time of visit<br>• required consultations | The decision to implement one or more of these strategies is a matter of clinical judgment. |
| Assess drug-related behaviors over time | Track drug use in tandem with all relevant outcomes. | Monitor drug-related behavior (eg, the need for early refills, obtaining multiple prescriptions, etc.).<br>Also monitor<br>• pain relief<br>• adverse drug effects<br>• effect of drug on other outcomes. | Broad monitoring of outcomes is consistent with integration of pain management into a palliative care model. |

Continued on page 76

Table 16. Principles of Risk Management During Opioid Therapy for Pain *(continued)*

| Principle | Goals | Strategies | Comment |
|---|---|---|---|
| Respond to aberrant drug-related behaviors | Clinician compliance with laws and regulations<br><br>Identifying patients needing additional management | If the patient engages in aberrant drug-related behavior, reassess and diagnose (addiction, other psychiatric disorder, pseudoaddiction, family issues, criminal intent)<br><br>If diversion into the illicit market is occurring, prescribing should cease. | Even advanced illness does not free clinicians from complying with laws and regulations. |
| Document and communicate | Risk assessment and management should be viewed as integral to safe and effective prescribing. | Document<br>• plan for monitoring and education of patients and families<br>• monitoring of drug-related behavior on a regular basis<br>• response if aberrant behavior occurs. | It is valuable to openly discuss the need for universal risk management with other clinicians to reduce the risk of stigmatizing patients. |

Reprinted from The Lancet, 377(9784), RK Portenoy, *Treatment of Cancer Pain*, 2236-2247, ©2011, with permission from Elsevier.

## Patients with Past or Current Substance Use Disorders

Treating pain for patients with past or current drug addictions presents special challenges, but treatment is possible[183,485,486] A multidisciplinary approach that includes a mental health provider who has experience with treating drug addiction can assist in both assessment and management of drug-related behavior. A detailed substance-use history is essential, and this should include information about social context, duration, frequency, specific drug preferences, and desired effect of drug use. It is important to set realistic goals for therapy. Patients should understand that safe and effective prescribing requires cessation of illicit drug use and increased adherence monitoring as prescribed controlled drugs are used. Comorbid psychiatric disorders including personality disorder, depression, and anxiety should be evaluated and addressed.

Physicians also should consider the therapeutic impact of tolerance. Because opioid abusers may be tolerant of medications prescribed, and this tolerance cannot be measured, it is recommended to start conservatively but to rapidly titrate the opioid dosage and reassess frequently for acute pain. If concerns about adherence or severe pain complicate the effort to manage drug titration, admission to a monitored setting may be the safest and best course of action.

Nonadherence behaviors or aberrant drug-related behaviors must be monitored for all patients prescribed opioid therapy (**Table 17**). For ambulatory patients, it is commonplace to obtain urine or saliva drug levels periodically during the course of therapy. If a patient has a history of significant drug abuse, this screening should be done when long-term opioid therapy is initiated and then periodically considered for repeat testing thereafter. Drug screening should be explained to the patient as a routine safety measure. This conversation need not suggest any lack of trust, but rather should provide the type of documentation necessary for physicians to act consistently in the patient's best interest. It is important to make use of statewide pharmacy databases to identify any prescriptions coming from other providers. Also, caution must be used when blending benzodiazepines with opioids because the combination of these two classes can increase the risk of inadvertent fatal overdose.

In some cases written statements (eg, a medication management or pain treatment agreement) that explain the roles of team members and the rules and expectations of the patient can be helpful, but they are controversial, and there is little evidence that they protect patients or physicians.[487] Patients with aberrant behavior should be seen more frequently and possibly referred to a specialist in addiction medicine.

## Opioids and Tolerance

*Tolerance* is a state of adaptation through which exposure to a drug induces changes that result in the diminished effects of a drug over time. Tolerance to analgesia, if it occurs, may be problematic, necessitating the use of higher dosages that may preclude effective pain management. Some clinicians are so concerned about analgesic tolerance they advocate "saving" the drug until life expectancy is short. This is inappropriate. Treatment-limiting analgesic tolerance is an unusual problem in the clinical setting. After an effective baseline dose is established, requirements usually plateau until the disease progresses, at which time the dosage is

## Table 17. Behaviors Suggestive of Addiction

**Behaviors Less Indicative of Addiction**

- Expressed anxiety or desperation over recurrent symptoms
- Hoarded medications
- Taken someone else's pain medication
- Aggressively complained to the doctor for more drugs
- Requested a specific drug or medication
- Used more opioids than the physician recommended
- Drinks more alcohol when in pain
- Expressed worry over changing to a new drug, even if the drug would have fewer side effects
- Raised opioid dose on their own
- Expressed concern to family, saying that pain might lead to use of street drugs
- Expressed concern to doctor, saying that pain might lead to use of street drugs
- Asked for a second opinion about pain medications
- Smoked cigarettes to relieve pain
- Used opioids to treat other symptoms

**Behaviors More Indicative of Addiction**

- Multiple prescribers of controlled substances
- Bought pain medication from a street dealer
- Stole money to obtain drugs
- Tried to get opioids from more than one source
- Performed sex for drugs
- Stole drugs from others
- Performed sex for money to obtain drugs
- Selling prescription drugs
- Prostituted others for money to obtain drugs
- Prostituted others for drugs
- Prescription forgery

*From SD Passik, KL Kirsh, KB Konaghy, and RK Portenoy, Pain and Aberrant Drug-Related Behaviors in Medically Ill Patients With and Without Histories of Substance Abuse, Clin J Pain, 22(2), 173-181, http:// journals.lww.com/clinicalpain/Abstract/2006/02000/Pain_and_Aberrant_Drug_Related_Behaviors_ in.9.aspx. ©2006 Lippincott Williams & Wilkins. Reproduced with permission.*

increased to control increased levels of pain. Opioids should be used when pain severity warrants this therapy and not be delayed because of concern about loss of efficacy over time.

### Opioids and Risk of Hastened Death

Clinicians may withhold opioid therapy to address ongoing pain because of concerns that the opioid drug will hasten death for patients with far-advanced illness who are likely to die in the near future. This is both a clinical and ethical challenge. Yes, opioid therapy can reduce respiratory reserve. Data from large observational studies are reassuring, however, and suggest that the influence of opioids on the timing of death is nil or minor in most cases.[488,489] Nevertheless, the possibility of hastening death or prolonging life cannot be entirely negated. Clinicians should have a solid understanding of the ethical basis for continuing effective opioid therapy in this context. Some clinicians refer to the ethical principle of double effect to provide a supportive framework and to help guide practice and educate others (see *UNIPAC 6*). Others solely rely on careful assessment of risks and benefits when recommending therapies intended for symptom relief and comfort in the terminal setting; these clinicians do not think that the principle of double effect is needed to justify treatment.

## Other Misconceptions

Lack of familiarity with long-term opioid therapy in medically ill populations may drive other misapprehensions that may be expressed by patients, family members, or professionals. Many people do not appreciate the extraordinary effective dose range of this drug class. Oral morphine, 2 mg every 4 hours, may be an effective dose for some patients, while others may require the equivalent of grams per day. Repeated dose escalation in an effort to identify and retain a favorable balance between analgesia and side effects is appropriate; the occurrence of treatment-limiting side effects defines poor responsiveness to the regimen and requires a change in therapy.

Another misconception relates to routes of administration. Some perceive that parenteral drugs are more effective than oral drugs. With opioid compounds, efficacy is related to dose, and in most cases equivalent analgesia between the oral and parenteral routes is possible with dose adjustment. The decision to employ parenteral therapy should be based on need, such as the need for rapid titration due to uncontrolled pain, treatment of incident breakthrough pain, or the need for more reliable absorption for patients with bowel obstruction or short gut syndrome.[490,491]

Some patients mistake itch and urticaria, known side effects of opioids, for a true allergy. Others perceive nausea in the same way. Although true allergic hypersensitivity can occur, such reactions are distinctly rare.

## Nonopioid Analgesics

Acetaminophen (also known as paracetamol) and NSAIDs comprise the nonopioid analgesic drugs available in the United States. The analgesic mechanism of acetaminophen is poorly understood but may involve inhibition of prostaglandin formation in the CNS. In contrast to NSAIDs, acetaminophen is not antiinflammatory. Given its favorable safety profile, it may be considered for the long-term treatment of mild pain, notwithstanding scant evidence that the combination of acetaminophen plus an opioid is more effective than an opioid alone.[492-495]

### Acetaminophen

Acetaminophen has a narrow therapeutic window. In the United States, concerns about unintentional overdose have been rising, and regulators are now limiting the amount of acetaminophen to 325 mg per dose, suggesting that a maximum dose should be 2.6 g per day (eight tablets per day of a formulation containing 325 mg per dose unit[496]). An underlying mechanism for acetaminophen toxicity may be glutathione deficiency.[497] Acetylcysteine has long been recognized as an effective antidote, via oral or intravenous administration, minimizing the risk and severity of acute liver injury if administered sufficiently early after an acetaminophen overdose. Despite this, its mechanisms of action remain obscure, and there is uncertainty regarding the optimal dose and duration of treatment.[498] Regulators suggest that patients with significant liver disease should be limited to 2 g to 3 g of acetaminophen daily, and if patients are abusing alcohol, it should not be used at all.[499] In addition, significant weight loss is associated with acetaminophen toxicity, which may be particularly important for patients with cachexia.[500]

## Nonsteroidal Antiinflammatory Drugs

NSAIDs comprise a diverse drug class (**Table 18**)[501] that produces analgesia by inhibiting the enzyme cyclooxygenase (COX) in the periphery and CNS, thereby reducing tissue levels of peripheral and central prostaglandins. There are two main forms of COX: a form that largely is constitutive (COX-1) and a form that largely is induced during the inflammatory cascade (COX-2). All NSAIDs inhibit both COX-1 and COX-2, but with varying selectivity.

NSAIDs have analgesic, antiinflammatory, and antipyretic effects. They are effective analgesics in combination with opioids[502,503] and may be especially useful for patients with bone pain or pain that is related to gross inflammatory lesions. They appear to be less useful for patients who have neuropathic pain.

A risk assessment will strongly influence the selection of patients with serious illness for a trial of NSAID therapy. The patient risk profile assessment is an essential step in the decision to try or withhold NSAID therapy.

All NSAIDs produce GI toxicity, which ranges from pain, nausea, or heartburn to ulceration and bleeding. Drugs that are more selective for COX-2 are relatively less likely to produce side effects related to COX-1 inhibition, such as GI toxicity. Drugs specifically developed as selective COX-2 inhibitors have been shown to produce fewer GI effects when low-dose aspirin therapy is not taken concurrently.[504] Limited data suggest that some of the nonselective NSAIDs (eg, ibuprofen, naproxen, nabumetone, the nonacetylated salicylates such as choline magnesium trisalicylate and salsalate) also pose a relatively lower risk for this toxicity.[505,506] Regardless of the drug, the risk of serious GI toxicity is higher in those older than 60 years, those with a history of an ulcer or GI hemorrhage, those receiving a corticosteroid or anticoagulant, and those receiving a high dose of the NSAID. H. pylori also may be a risk factor, and patients with a history of gastritis or ulcer disease can be tested for this infection. NSAIDs should be considered relatively contraindicated in patients with multiple risk factors. Those with only one or two risk factors should be strongly considered for treatment with a selective COX-2 inhibitor (celecoxib) or a coadministered gastroprotective drug, usually a proton-pump inhibitor.[507]

All NSAIDs also produce cardiovascular toxicities, which include fluid retention (associated with blood pressure elevation and risk of volume overload) and prothrombotic effects. The prothrombotic effect, which appears to be related to inhibition of the COX-2 enzyme, predisposes to angina and myocardial infarction, transient ischemic attack and stroke, and symptomatic peripheral vascular disease.[504] Mostly because of the latter concern, two COX-2 selective NSAIDs were taken off the US market, and others have not been approved. Subsequent research has concluded that cardiovascular toxicity characterizes all NSAIDs, and there is large drug-related variation in this risk.[508] Indeed, the only labeled COX-2 selective drug in the United States, celecoxib, appears to pose a far lower risk than other drugs in this class; similarly, some of the nonselective drugs such as naproxen and ibuprofen appear to present relatively lower risk for these cardiovascular events.

With the exception of the nonacetylated salicylates (choline magnesium trisalicylate and salsalate) and the selective COX-2 inhibitors (celecoxib), all NSAIDs interfere with platelet aggregation. Despite its short half-life, aspirin irreversibly inhibits platelet aggregation for the lifetime of the platelet (4-7 days). The inhibitory effect of other NSAIDs lasts about 2 days. NSAID therapy generally is avoided for patients with a bleeding diathesis of any type.

All NSAIDS can adversely affect renal function. The range of potential lesions is large and includes acute interstitial nephritis, acute tubular necrosis in patients with low renal perfusion, and chronic nephropathy. NSAIDs also should be avoided in patients who are dehydrated, have renal insufficiency, or have disorders associated with a high likelihood of renal dysfunction (eg, multiple myeloma).

Significant hepatotoxicity from NSAID therapy is uncommon, but mild elevations in liver enzymes are frequently encountered. In the context of serious illness, stable and mild elevations should be monitored over time; the drug may be continued if it is providing benefit.

Considering this range of toxicities, the decision to offer a trial of NSAID treatment should take into account the likelihood of benefit and the risk of adverse effects as well as the cost and burden associated with prolonged treatment. Risk profiling should inform drug selection, which in most cases would begin with one of the drugs known to pose a relatively lower risk for GI toxicity (eg, celecoxib) or a drug with relatively low cardiovascular toxicity (naproxen).[506,508] Regardless of the drug selected, lower doses are associated with less risk than higher doses. Most patients have one or more risk factors for GI toxicity, so concurrent use of a gastroprotective drug such as omeprazole also can be considered.

Because there is substantial variability in patient response to various NSAIDs, the decision to try an NSAID may require several trials to identify the agent with the most favorable risk-to-benefit ratio. Past response to an NSAID may inform current drug selection, and pharmacokinetic considerations (eg, use of a drug with once-daily or twice-daily administration) also may be important.

## Table 18. NSAIDs and Related Analgesics[501]

| Generic Name | Approximate Half-Life (Hours) | Starting Daily Dosage | Maximum Daily Dosage | Excretion | Comments* |
|---|---|---|---|---|---|
| **Para-Aminophenol Derivatives** | | | | | |
| Acetaminophen | 2-4 | 650-1,000 mg every 4-6 hours PO or IV | 4,000 mg | 85% renal | Lacks peripheral anti-inflammatory and anti-platelet effect. Excessive dosing leads to liver toxicity. Monitor platelet and liver function with chronic disease. |
| **Nonsteroidal Antiinflammatory Analgesics** | | | | | |
| *Salicylates* | | | | | |
| Acetylsalicylic acid (aspirin) | 3-12 | 325-650 mg every 4 hours | 6,000 mg | 100% renal | May inhibit platelet aggregation for > 1 week. Contraindicated for children with fever or other viral syndromes. |
| Choline magnesium trisalicylate | 8-12 | Initial dose: 1,500 mg, then 1,500 mg every 8-12 hours; 750 mg every 8-12 hours for older patients | 4,500 mg | 100% renal | Approved for children Minimal GI toxicity Suspension available Minimal platelet effects |
| Diflunisal | 8-12 | Initial dose: 1,000 mg, then 500 mg every 12 hours | 1,500 mg | 90% renal, < 5% fecal | N/A |
| Salsalate | 8-12 | Initial dose: 1,500 mg, then 1,500 mg every 12 hours | 3,000 mg | 100% renal | Minimal platelet effects |

## Table 18. NSAIDs and Related Analgesics[501] (continued)

| Generic Name | Approximate Half-Life (Hours) | Starting Daily Dosage | Maximum Daily Dosage | Excretion | Comments* |
|---|---|---|---|---|---|
| **Propionic Acids** | | | | | |
| Flurbiprofen | 5-6 | 50-100 mg every 6-8 hours | 300 mg | 65%-85% renal | N/A |
| Ibuprofen | 2-4 | 400-600 mg every 6-8 hours | 3,200 mg | 50%-75% renal | Suspension formulation available |
| Ketoprofen | 2-4 | 75 mg every 8 hours or 50 mg every 6 hours; 25-50 mg every 8 hours for mild renal impairment and older patients | 300 mg | 50%-90% renal, 1%-8% fecal | N/A |
| Naproxen | 13 | Initial dose: 500 mg, then 250 mg every 6-8 hours | 1,500 mg | 95% renal | Cautious use of > 1,500 mg/day may be more efficacious. Suspension available. |
| Oxaprozin | 50-60; 40 with repeated dosing | 1,200 mg daily | 1,800 mg | 60% renal, 30%-35% fecal | N/A |
| **Acetic Acids** | | | | | |
| Diclofenac | 2 | 50 mg every 8-12 hours | 150 mg | 50%-70% renal, 30%-35% fecal | A 1% topical gel is available for osteoarthritis. |

Continued on page 84

## Table 18. NSAIDs and Related Analgesics[501] (continued)

| Generic Name | Approximate Half-Life (Hours) | Starting Daily Dosage | Maximum Daily Dosage | Excretion | Comments* |
|---|---|---|---|---|---|
| Indomethacin | 4-5 | 25-50 mg every 8-12 hours | 200 mg | 60% renal, 30% fecal | Available in sustained release and rectal formulations. Greater GI and CNS toxicity. Not recommended for older patients. |
| Sulindac | 8-16 | 150 mg every 12 hours | 400 mg | 50% renal, 25% fecal | N/A |
| Tolmetin | 1 | 400 mg every 8 hours | 1,800 mg | 100% renal | N/A |
| Piroxicam | 50 | 20 mg daily | 20 mg | 67% renal, 33% fecal | Progressive increase in response may occur because of long half-life; steady state 7-12 days after initiation of therapy |
| Meclofenamic acid | 50 minutes-3.3 hours | 50-100 mg every 4-6 hours | 400 mg | 67% renal, 20%-25% fecal | Dose-related diarrhea |
| Mefenamic acid | 2 | Loading dose: 500 mg, then 250 mg every 6 hours | 1,000 mg | 67% renal, 33% fecal | Intended for short-term use; dose-related diarrhea |
| *COX-2 Inhibitors* | | | | | |
| Celecoxib | 11 | 100 mg twice daily; can give 400 mg on first day of administration | 200 mg after first day of administration | 97% hepatic metabolism, 3% renal | Less GI toxicity Increased cardiovascular events Minimal platelet Be aware of sulfa allergy |

## Table 18. NSAIDs and Related Analgesics[501] (continued)

| Generic Name | Approximate Half-Life (Hours) | Starting Daily Dosage | Maximum Daily Dosage | Excretion | Comments* |
|---|---|---|---|---|---|
| **Pyrrolizine** | | | | | |
| Ketorolac | 4-6 | IV/IM: 30 mg every 6 hours; 15 mg every 6 hours for older patients PO: 10 mg every 4-6 hours | IV/IM: 120 mg; 60 mg for older patients PO: 40 mg | 91% renal, 6% fecal | Usually used as single dose IV/IM. Maximum duration is 5 days. |
| **Pyranocarboxylic Acids** | | | | | |
| Etodolac | 6-7 | 200-400 mg every 6-8 hours | 1,200 mg | 60% renal, 27% fecal | N/A |
| **Naphthylalkanones** | | | | | |
| Nabumetone | 23-30 | 1,000 mg | 2,000 mg | Renal | N/A |

BUN, blood urea nitrogen; CNS, central nervous system; CV, cardiovascular; GI, gastrointestinal; IM, intramuscular; IV, intravenous; PO, by mouth.

* Use the lowest effective dosage for the shortest possible duration; see warnings below and as published for each drug.

Starting and maximal dosages are not intended to preclude clinical judgment of the prescriber. A dosage reduction is recommended for elderly patients, those with renal insufficiency, and when multiple medications are taken. Dosages can be incremented weekly. Studies of NSAIDs in the cancer population are limited. Dosing guidelines are based on studies in inflammatory diseases; consequently, dosages in patients with cancer are empiric.

NSAIDs can cause severe or life-threatening CV, GI, and renal toxicities, especially in older and chronically ill patients or if prescribed at high dosages over longer periods. If they must be used under high-risk circumstances, consider regular monitoring of stools for occult blood and BUN, creatinine, and liver function.

## Adjuvant Analgesics

The term *adjuvant analgesic* originally was coined to refer to a small number of drugs that were marketed for indications other than pain but were found to be potentially useful as analgesics in patients receiving opioid therapy. During the past 3 decades, the number, diversity, and uses of these drugs have increased dramatically, and several now are indicated as first-line therapy for certain types of pain.[509] As a result, the term, *adjuvant analgesic* has become somewhat of a misnomer, but it still is commonly applied in the context of cancer pain. The term is used interchangeably with *coanalgesic*.

Adjuvant analgesics can be used early but are often considered when pain has a relatively poor response to opioids (defined as the inability to maintain analgesia without producing significant side effects). The addition of an adjuvant analgesic is one approach among many that may be considered for such patients.[510] With the exception of certain pain states for which specific drugs have been identified as potential first-line therapies, a trial of a coanalgesic usually should be considered only after efforts have been made to optimize opioid therapy.

The large and growing number of adjuvant analgesics (**Table 19**) can be categorized on the basis of how they are used in clinical practice.[509] Based on conventional practice, the categories of available agents include

- drugs potentially useful for any type of pain (multipurpose analgesics)
- drugs used to treat neuropathic pain
- drugs used for bone pain
- drugs used for pain and other symptoms in the setting of bowel obstruction
- drugs specifically formulated for primary headache disorders.

### Multipurpose Analgesics

Some drug classes have been studied in diverse types of chronic pain, including corticosteroids, antidepressants, alpha-2 adrenergic agonists, cannabinoids, and topical therapies (Table 19). These drugs have broad indications.

### Glucocorticoids

In palliative care, corticosteroids are used to address pain, nausea, fatigue, anorexia, and malaise.[511-513] Based on extensive observations, these drugs may be analgesic for neuropathic and bone pain, pain associated with capsular expansion or duct obstruction, pain from bowel obstruction, pain caused by lymphedema, and headache caused by increased intracranial pressure. The mechanism of analgesia probably relates to reduction of tumor-related edema, antiinflammatory effects, and direct effects on pain pathways.

Dexamethasone is usually preferred, presumably because of its long half-life and relatively low mineralocorticoid effects. There is no evidence, however, that this drug is safer or more effective than other corticosteroids. A typical regimen is 1 mg to 2 mg of dexamethasone orally or parenterally once or twice daily; this may be preceded by a larger loading dose of 10 mg to 20 mg. This regimen, or comparable regimens of alternative steroids, is based

## Table 19. Adjuvant Analgesics

| Drug Class | Subclass | Examples | Comments |
|---|---|---|---|
| **Multipurpose Analgesics** | | | |
| Glucocorticoids | N/A | Dexamethasone, prednisone | Used for bone pain, neuropathic pain, lymphedema pain, headache, bowel obstruction |
| Antidepressants | Tricyclics | Desipramine, amitriptyline | Used for opioid-refractory neuropathic pain first if comorbid depression; secondary amine compounds (eg, desipramine, nortriptyline) have fewer side effects and may be preferred |
| | SNRIs | Duloxetine, venlafaxine | Good evidence in some conditions but overall less than tricyclics; however, better side-effect profile; often tried first |
| | SSRIs | Paroxetine, citalopram | Very limited evidence, and if pain is the target, other subclasses preferred |
| | Other | Bupropion | Limited evidence but less sedating, and often tried early when fatigue or somnolence is a problem |
| Alpha-2 adrenergic agonists | N/A | Tizanidine, clonidine | Seldom used systemically because of side effects, but tizanidine is preferred for a trial; clonidine is used in neuraxial analgesia |
| Cannabinoid | N/A | THC/cannabidiol, nabilone, THC | Good evidence in cancer pain for THC/cannabidiol; limited evidence for other commercially available compounds |
| Topical agents | Anesthetic | Lidocaine patch, local anesthetic creams | N/A |
| | Capsaicin | 8% patch; 0.25%, 0.75% creams | High-concentration patch indicated for postherpetic neuralgia |
| | NSAIDs | Diclofenac and others | Evidence in focal musculoskeletal pains |
| | Tricyclics | Doxepin cream | Used in itch; may be tried for pain |
| | Other | Compounded creams with varied drugs tried empirically, but no evidence |

Continued on page 88

## Table 19. Adjuvant Analgesics (continued)

| Drug Class | Subclass | Examples | Comments |
|---|---|---|---|
| **Used for Neuropathic Pain** | | | |
| Multipurpose drugs | As above | As above | As above |
| Anticonvulsants | Gabapentinoids | Gabapentin, pregabalin | Used first for opioid-refractory neuropathic pain unless comorbid depression; may be multipurpose considering evidence in postsurgical pain; both drugs act at the N-type calcium channel in the CNS, but response to one or the other varies |
| | Other | Oxcarbazepine, lamotrigine, topiramate, lacosamide, divalproex, carbamazepine, phenytoin | Limited evidence for all examples listed; newer drugs preferred because of less side-effect liability, but individual variation is wide; all are considered for opioid-refractory neuropathic pain if antidepressants and gabapentinoids are ineffective |
| Sodium channel drugs | Sodium channel blockers | Mexiletine, IV lidocaine | Good evidence for IV lidocaine |
| | Sodium channel modulator | Lacosamide | New anticonvulsant with limited evidence of analgesic effects |
| GABA agonists | GABA$_A$ agonist | Clonazepam | Limited evidence, but used for neuropathic pain with anxiety |
| | GABA$_B$ agonist | Baclofen | Evidence in trigeminal neuralgia is the basis for trials in other types of neuropathic pain |

**Table 19. Adjuvant Analgesics** *(continued)*

| Drug Class | Subclass | Examples | Comments |
|---|---|---|---|
| N-methyl-D-aspartate inhibitors | N/A | Ketamine, memantine, others | Limited evidence for ketamine, but positive experience for IV use in advanced illness or a pain crisis; little evidence for oral drugs |
| **Used for Bone Pain** | | | |
| Bisphospho-nates | N/A | Pamidronate, ibandronate, clodronate | Good evidence; like the NSAIDs or glucocorticoids, usually considered first-line therapy; also reduces other adverse skeletal-related events; concern about osteonecrosis of the jaw and renal insufficiency; may limit use |
| Calcitonin | N/A | N/A | Limited evidence but usually well-tolerated |
| Radiopharma-ceuticals | N/A | Strontium-89, samarium-153 | Good evidence, but limited use because of bone marrow effects and need for expertise |
| **Used for Bowel Obstruction** | | | |
| Anticholinergic drugs | N/A | Scopolamine (hyoscine) compounds, glycopyrrolate | Along with a glucocorticoid, considered first-line adjuvant for nonsurgical bowel obstruction |
| Somatostatin analogue | N/A | Octreotide | Along with a glucocorticoid, considered first-line adjuvant for nonsurgical bowel obstruction |

*CNS, central nervous system; GABA, gamma-aminobutyric acid; IV, intravenous; NSAID, nonsteroidal antiinflammatory drug; SNRI, -serotonin norepinephrine reuptake inhibitor; SSRI, selective serotonin reuptake inhibitor; THC, tetrahydrocannabinol.*

*Reprinted from The Lancet, 377(9784), RK Portenoy, Treatment of Cancer Pain, 2236-2247, ©2011, with permission from Elsevier.*

on clinical experience. Patients may do well with lower or higher doses or with once-daily rather than twice-daily dosing. Very high dose therapy (eg, dexamethasone, 50 mg to 100 mg intravenously, followed by 12 mg to 24 mg four times daily, tapered over 1-3 weeks) has been used empirically for pain crises related to bone or nerve injury. This approach was developed for treatment of emerging spinal cord compression and has been observed to yield rapid pain relief with acceptable risk of adverse effects.[514]

Long-term corticosteroid therapy may produce myopathy, worsening immunosuppression, psychotomimetic effects, and hypoadrenalism. These risks must be balanced against the observed benefit.

## Analgesic Antidepressants

Antidepressants have been widely studied as analgesics for varied types of chronic pain.[509,515-518] Although very few of these studies have included medically ill patients, the utility of these drugs in these populations is accepted. In opioid-treated populations with advanced medical illness, these drugs usually are considered for patients with refractory neuropathic pain.

Antidepressants produce analgesia independently of mood effects. Pain reduction may be enhanced, however, if there is a concurrent positive mood effect. The analgesic mode of action is thought to be related to enhanced availability of monoamines in descending pain-modulating systems. Inhibition of norepinephrine reuptake appears to be the most important mode of action, but serotonergic and dopaminergic effects probably play a role in analgesia.

Antidepressants may be categorized by subclasses. Analgesic efficacy is best established for some of the tricyclic compounds[515,519-521] and the serotonin-norepinephrine reuptake inhibitors (SNRIs)[518,521-524]; there is minimal evidence of analgesic efficacy with SSRIs.[515,525,526] There also is limited evidence for bupropion, a dopamine reuptake inhibitor.[527]

Tricyclic antidepressants include tertiary amines such as amitriptyline and the secondary amines nortriptyline and desipramine. Secondary amines are more selective at noradrenergic reuptake sites and have a more favorable side effect profile than amitriptyline, but both desipramine and nortriptyline have weak evidence for analgesic benefit relative to amitriptyline[528,529] All tricyclic compounds are relatively contraindicated for patients with serious heart disease, severe prostatic hypertrophy, and narrow-angle glaucoma.

There is strong evidence that duloxetine, an SNRI, is analgesic.[523,524] There is less evidence for others in this class, including milnacipran, venlafaxine, and desvenlafaxine. The side effect profile of this class includes nausea, sexual dysfunction, and somnolence or mental clouding. Side effects usually are less limiting for this class of antidepressant than for secondary amine tricyclics, but there is a great deal of individual variation. Among patients with serious medical illness, the first-line analgesic antidepressants may be either one of the secondary amine tricyclic compounds (usually desipramine) or duloxetine, and the decision between these drugs usually is based on a case-by-case assessment of risk and cost.

Other antidepressants usually are considered only if first-line antidepressants are ineffective. The exception is bupropion, which is a dopamine and norepinephrine reuptake inhibitor

## Refractory Constipation

Patients with refractory constipation may be considered for other therapies; most important among these is the peripherally acting opioid antagonist methylnaltrexone.[366,373] A recent metaanalysis demonstrated an increased likelihood of producing a rescue-free bowel movement within 4 hours of administration of methylnaltrexone as compared with placebo. Effective doses were 0.3 mg/kg every other day or 12 mg per day, both by injection.[374] Three doses (daily or every other day) may be needed to judge the benefits. Patients who have not responded to the treatment after three doses are unlikely to respond. Adverse reactions include abdominal pain, usually described as "cramps," that is generally mild to moderate in severity and decreases in incidence with subsequent dosing.[375] Other peripherally acting antagonists are in development, and oral naloxone also may be used.[142,146] Alvimopan, an oral agent, is approved for postoperative use in hospitalized patients via a limited-access program, but it also has been effective for patients with OIC.[376] Opioid antagonists should be considered only when the presence of mechanical obstruction has been excluded. Lubiprostone is labeled for OIC. It is a chloride channel stimulating laxative.[377-379] Nausea, cramps, and diarrhea are reported side effects. Costs may be an issue, particularly for hospices. Naloxegol has recently been approved to treat OIC experienced by patients with noncancer pain.[380] It is only approved for OIC experienced by patients with noncancer pain and is likely, at the present time, to not be covered by insurance. Linaclotide, another enteric chloride channel stimulant, is being studied in patients with OIC.[381]

## Severe Constipation

Rectal suppositories and enemas are needed when a laxative regimen is conscientiously followed and fails to produce laxation. These approaches are used if severe constipation and nausea develop. Oral laxatives should not be used if there is a bowel obstruction; enemas or suppositories may be used to treat a suspected low impaction. Impactions may better respond to mineral oil or cottonseed oil to soften the hard stool. Mineral oil should not be used by mouth. Aspiration of mineral oil can cause a severe pneumonitis.[382-384] Rectal bisacodyl (one to two suppositories) or high-volume enemas may be considered along with aggressive oral therapies such as sorbitol, lactulose, or polyethylene glycol two to six times daily until a bowel movement occurs.

## *Nausea and Vomiting*

The nausea and vomiting associated with opioids is more difficult to manage than OIC.[385] The emetogenic reflexes are transmitted via the vagus through the area postrema (a circumventricular organ in the medulla that does not have a blood brain barrier) and nucleus tractus solitarius. The region of the area postrema and the nucleus tractus solitarius is called the chemoreceptor trigger zone. The chemoreceptor trigger zone projects to the vomiting center, a group of neurons within the medulla that becomes a central pattern generator for emesis. The vomiting center receives input not only from the chemoreceptor trigger zone but also vestibular apparatus and cerebral cortex. Opioids produce emesis in several ways: (a) inhibition of gut motility, (b) binding to mu receptors within the chemoreceptor trigger zone, and (c) stimulating the vestibular apparatus.[386] Several different causes for nausea and vomiting may occur with a single individual, making it difficult to determine how much the opioid therapy contributes to nausea and vomiting. Constipation, other medications, intraabdominal or brain metastases, pain, vestibular diseases, and anxiety may contribute to nausea and vomiting while someone is receiving opioid therapy.[36] What once was assumed to be opioid-induced nausea and vomiting may in fact be related to the above-mentioned factors. There is rapid tolerance to opioid-induced nausea and vomiting. Mu receptors within the vomiting center when activated are actually antiemetic, whereas mu receptors within the chemoreceptor trigger zone cause nausea and vomiting when activated.[387-390] However, a subgroup of individuals will have persistent nausea and vomiting and do not appear to develop tolerance.[391] Opioid dose titration can lead to a resurgence of nausea and emesis. This also can occur as a "bolus" effect from a rescue opioid dose.

The incidence of nausea and vomiting differs between opioids.[392] Metoclopramide reduces nausea caused by gastric stasis and blocks dopamine receptors centrally, so theoretically it is a good choice. However, in a randomized trial, metoclopramide was no better than placebo in reducing opioid-induced nausea.[393] The same was true for ondansetron. Both histamine receptor antagonists and anticholinergics have been reported to improve opioid-induced nausea and vomiting in nonrandomized trials. Scopolamine patches have been used with some effect but have not been tested in randomized trials.[394] In a small retrospective study, risperidone did reduce nausea and vomiting related to opioids.[395] For children, small doses of naloxone (dosages lower than that which reverses analgesia) can reduce nausea and vomiting from opioids.[396] Management includes ruling out other causes of nausea and vomiting. Opioid dose reduction or rotation have proven to be beneficial in a significant number of patients.[397,398]

## Musculoskeletal Adverse Events
Opioids are associated with an increased risk of falls and fractures for older people. This may be due to dizziness and reduced alertness.[399] This adverse effect occurs early in the course of opioid therapy. The relative risk for a fall with a resulting fracture for older patients is 1.4 relative to people not taking opioids. However, the hazard ratio can be as high as 4.9 compared with matched controls on NSAIDs.[400] Morphine dosages greater than 50 mg per day double the fracture risk for older patients. The annual rate of fracture is as high as 10%.[401-403] Buprenorphine is not associated with a risk for falls.[404] Short-acting opioids may lead to a greater risk for fracture than long-acting opioids, particularly within the first 2 weeks of initiating opioid therapy.[405]

## Osteoporosis
Long-term opioid therapy is associated with osteoporosis. In a study involving individuals on maintenance opioids for addiction, 74% had a low bone mass. This was irrespective of the opioid used in maintenance therapy. For those older than 40 years, 29% had osteoporosis (T score -3.0) and 48% had osteopenia (T score -1.7). Most men younger than 40 years (66%)

that is distinguished by the tendency to be mentally activating. A trial of bupropion sometimes is considered early on if pain is complicated by somnolence, even though the evidence of analgesia is weak.

All of the analgesic antidepressants should be started at relatively low initial doses. The starting dose for desipramine is 10 mg to 25 mg at night. The dose should be increased slowly until pain improves or side effects occur. The long half-life of tricyclics (24 hours) means that doses are given once daily, preferably at night, and increased slowly at 5- to 7-day intervals. The usual effective antidepressant dose of desipramine is between 50 mg and 150 mg per day. Other antidepressants such as duloxetine or bupropion should similarly be started at a relatively low initial dose and titrated to conventional maximal doses to determine whether an analgesic or positive mood effect occurs. Doses of these antidepressants are best given in the morning. Duloxetine may be started at 30 mg daily and increased to 60 mg 1 week later.

In clinical practice, lower doses of the tricyclic drugs are used for pain and sleep (eg, desipramine, 25 mg-75 mg at bedtime). At relatively high doses of a tricyclic drug (> 100 mg/day) the plasma drug concentration and an electrocardiogram should be checked. Tricyclic antidepressants can prolong the QTc interval and predispose to cardiac arrhythmias. These drugs should be used cautiously when a patient has known heart disease or is receiving other drugs that can prolong the QTc interval, such as methadone.

## Alpha-2 Adrenergic Agonists

Clonidine, which can be administered by oral, transdermal, or intraspinal routes, has been studied in patients with chronic noncancer pain and was shown to be analgesic for both neuropathic and nociceptive pain in a controlled cancer pain trial.[530] There is less evidence of analgesic efficacy with oral tizanidine[531] and parenteral dexmedetomidine.[532] These drugs can produce somnolence and dry mouth and may cause hypotension. Considering these side effects and limited evidence of benefit, they seldom are used systemically for pain in medically ill populations. For those with refractory neuropathic pain or muscle spasm, tizanidine (which has less hypotensive effect than clonidine) may be considered for a cautious trial.

## Cannabinoids

Cannabinoids not only bind to classical receptors (CB1 and CB2) but also to certain orphan receptors (GPR-55 and GPR-119) and ion channels (transient receptor potential) in medically ill populations.[533] The CB1 receptor is responsible for the psychotomimetic effects associated with tetrahydrocannabinol (THC). The second most common cannabinoid in phytocannabinoids is cannabidiol (CBD), which is a CB1 receptor antagonist. Cannabinoids appear to have an "entourage" when combined and either improve responses such as analgesia or reduce side effects, hence the rationale for combining THC and CBD.[534] Cannabinoids are known to modulate a multitude of monoamine receptors. Multiple studies, most of which are of moderate to low quality, demonstrate that tetrahydrocannabinol and oromucosal cannabinoid combinations of THC and CBD modestly reduce cancer pain. See *UNIPAC 4*, Anorexia-Cachexia chapter, for discussion of the use of cannabinoids for appetite stimulation.

## A Summary of Key Cannabinoid Studies

Two studies published in 1975 compared dronabinol to placebo for cancer pain. Dronabinol, 10 mg daily, was better tolerated than 20 mg. Side effects were dizziness, somnolence, ataxia, and blurred vision. Analgesia was modest and equivalent to 60 mg and 120 mg of oral codeine, respectively.[535,536]

A systematic review of cannabinoids for pain found a small benefit for cannabinoids (standard mean difference in pain was -0.61 on a 0-10 NRS [95% CI, -0.37 to -0.84]). Cannabinoids were much more likely to result in adverse effects (OR, 4.5; 95% CI, 3.0-6.6), including altered perception and impaired psychomotor and cognitive function.[537]

Two recent trials have used nabiximols, which is an oromucosal spray containing 2.7 mg THC and 2.5 mg CBD per 100 mcL. Individuals were on 271 mg daily morphine equivalent doses. The average dose was 8.75 sprays per day (24 mg THC). The difference in pain severity by NRS was -0.67 ($P$ = .014); adjusted differences between groups were -.055 ($P$ = .024). The 30% responder rate and the number needed to treat (NNT; the number of individuals needed to treat to reduce pain severity in one individual by 30%) was 43% with nabiximols and 21% with the placebo (NNT = 4.7). No pain relief was seen at THC doses greater than 22.5 mg per day.[538]

The second trial involved four groups of patients: placebo, low dose (1-4 sprays per day), medium-dose (6-10 sprays per day), and high-dose (11-16 sprays per day) nabiximols. The median morphine daily equivalent for the group was 120 mg. This study failed to meet the primary outcome of 30% reduction in pain severity. Some benefit was noted in reduction of pain severity in the lower and medium-dose groups but not in the high-dose group (-0.75 with the low dose, -.036 with the medium dose).[539] This study, like the first study, demonstrated a dose ceiling effect with pain. There was some improvement in sleep but also an increase in nausea with nabiximols at the high dose.

Nabiximols (2.7 mg/2.5 mg) also was investigated in an extension of two randomized trials involving patients with neuropathic pain. Up to 24 doses per day were used.[540] Individuals were kept on their prestudy analgesics. Two hundred thirty-four patients completed the study. Patients who had previously been on a placebo in the randomized trial had a discontinuation rate of 27%, and those who had received an active drug had an 11% discontinuation rate; discontinuation was largely because of adverse effects. Pain intensity by NRS decreased from 5.5 (0-10) to 4.2 over the 9-month period. Twenty-eight percent were responders (greater than or equal to 30% reduction in pain intensity). Approximately 75% reported some improvement in pain intensity, 22% had no change, and 8% worsened. Doses on average were 6-8 sprays per day. Maximum response occurred between weeks 14 and 26, and by week 38 pain began to increase, suggesting some analgesic tolerance. Sleep quality and QOL, which had improved on the randomized trial, were maintained in the open label study.[540]

### Topical Therapies

The most widely used topical therapies for pain contain local anesthetics. Lidocaine 5% patches[541] and various anesthetic gels or creams[542,543] may be applied to focal areas of pain related to nerve injury[544] or joint or soft tissue injury,[545] with the intent of producing analgesia. For the lidocaine patch, limited data indicate a high level of safety when four patches are applied within 24 hours and for up to 72 hours.[546] Long-term therapy with this number of patches or fewer may be considered.

Capsaicin, a naturally occurring compound in chili pepper, depletes substance P from the terminals of afferent C-fibers. Topical application of a low-concentration cream (0.1%) potentially can benefit patients with various types of neuropathic and joint pain.[547] Burning, which usually is transitory, is the major side effect. Application three to four times daily on a scheduled, not as-needed, basis for a period of at least 1 week is needed to determine benefit. In 2009 the FDA approved a high-concentration capsaicin patch (8%) for treatment of postherpetic neuralgia.[548] This patch is applied for 1 hour in a monitored environment and, if effective, can yield benefit for months. Local anesthetic is often applied to the area before the patch is applied.

Numerous antiinflammatory drugs have been investigated for topical use, and diclofenac, ibuprofen, and ketoprofen patch, cream, and gel have been studied in a large number of patients with acute musculoskeletal pain. Topical diclofenac has measured analgesia with an effect size by NNT of 3.7. Ketoprofen success by NNT is 3.9, as is topical ibuprofen. Local skin reactions occur in 4.3% of people.[549] The advantages to topical therapy are that the effects are local with less than 10% of the drug reaching systemic circulation. This reduces the risk of adverse events, particularly for older patients. Although studied in musculoskeletal pain,[550] there is favorable anecdotal experience in diverse types of pain.

Topical tricyclic antidepressants have been used as an analgesic,[551] and a doxepin cream is commercially available. Doxepin cream is indicated for pruritus but may be considered for patients with local or regional pain, especially neuropathic painful itch.

Other drugs have been compounded into creams for patients with pain. Medications for which there are published trials are ketamine, amitriptyline, and gabapentin, but a variety of others have been reported, including topical opioids. Supporting data for these therapies are meager or nonexistent, but topical application is generally safe. In the setting of refractory pain, a trial may be reasonable if cost is not prohibitive.

## Drugs Used for Neuropathic Pain

All of the multipurpose analgesics have been used for opioid-refractory neuropathic pain in medically ill people.[237] The SNRI and tricyclic antidepressants are widely considered as first-line for this indication if pain is accompanied by depressed mood.[552] Other first-line drugs for neuropathic pain are anticonvulsants, specifically the gabapentinoids.

### Gabapentinoids

Gabapentinoids (gabapentin and pregabalin) were initially designed as gamma-amino butyric acid (GABA) agonists. Both agents are lipophilic and quickly penetrate the CNS. In 1993 gabapentin was initially licensed for partial seizures for individuals younger than 12 years. However, in 2004, it was approved for postherpetic neuralgia. Gabapentin has been found to counter opioid-induced hyperalgesia.[229]

Pregabalin was developed as a successor to gabapentin. Pregabalin was licensed for the treatment of partial seizures in 2001 but subsequently was approved for treatment of painful diabetic neuropathy, and in Europe it is approved for anxiety disorders.[553,554] Later it was discovered that neither drug binds to, modulates, or influences GABA receptors nor does either drug influence GABA uptake, synthesis, or metabolism.[555,556]

Both gabapentin and pregabalin block the expression of the calcium channel alpha (2), delta-1 subunit expression on plasma membranes. The alpha (2), delta-1 subunit is upregulated in surviving neurons after neuropathic injury. Increased expression of calcium channels in plasma membrane surfaces increases neurotransmitter release.[557] There also appears to be a mechanism independent of calcium channels that produces pain relief before calcium channels are blocked.[557] Gabapentinoids produced an acute reduction in pain in human subjects who were given intradermal capsaicin to mimic neuropathic pain. The median single-dose response for pregabalin was 252 mg (95% CI, 194 mg-310 mg).[558] The single dose reduced tactile and thermal allodynia and secondary hyperalgesia around the area of capsaicin injury. Side effects to this high single dose were sedation (46%), euphoria (31%), and dizziness (7%).[558] Although high single-dose pregabalin has not been further tested in a well-designed trial, it should be explored further to determine how quickly one might respond with acute pain. Given this sedation effect, a single high dose at bedtime may both reduce severe acute neuropathic pain and allow patients to sleep. This approach has been reported to result in a quick response without a risk for respiratory depression. Similarly, single moderate doses of gabapentinoids have been demonstrated to reduce postoperative pain and opioid requirements. Appropriate dose titration can follow, beginning the next day, with anticipation of a clinical benefit. This may prevent the frustration of weeks of gabapentinoid titration without a response or waiting days to weeks to see a reduction in pain intensity.

Gabapentin requires a neutral amino transporter in the GI tract for absorption. Gabapentin is not absorbed per rectum for this reason. The transporter is saturable such that a lesser proportion of the drug is bioavailable at higher dosages. Unlike gabapentin, pregabalin is well-absorbed (> 90%) and absorption is independent of dose. Elimination of both gabapentinoids is unchanged in urine. Neither agent interacts with cytochromes and neither one is metabolized in the liver, hence there are few drug interactions.[559] Starting doses for gabapentin are 300 mg on day one, 600 mg on day two, and 900 mg on day three, with additional titration up to 1,800 mg. Dosages up to 3,600 mg daily may be needed. Dosages need to be divided into 8-hour increments.[560] Doses of pregabalin are 50 mg to 200 mg three times daily. Common adverse effects of gabapentinoids are somnolence, dizziness, gait disturbances, and edema.[556] In addition, pregabalin has a rewarding effect and is used to potentiate the rewarding effects and euphoria of opioids, which creates a potential for misuse and abuse.[561-563]

A summary of the benefits of gabapentinoids was published in 2015. The substantial improvement (50% reduction in pain intensity) for gabapentin when treating postherpetic neuralgia was 34% compared with 21% for placebo, an NNT of 8; and for diabetic neuropathy, 38% versus 21% for placebo with an NNT of 5.9. For all clinical trials, including those for other causes of neuropathic pain, the NNT was 7.2. Withdrawal for adverse effects was higher than placebo with a relative risk of 1.25. However, the number needed to treat to harm a single patient (NNH; withdrawal from the gabapentin) was 25.6, demonstrating a wide therapeutic index (NNH/NNT).[564] It does appear that if pain does not respond to one of the gabapentinoids, pain responses can occur with the alternative gabapentinoid.[565]

**Other Anticonvulsants**

Many other anticonvulsants have been studied as analgesics and may be considered for trials if opioid-refractory neuropathic pain does not respond to gabapentinoids or analgesic antidepressants.[566] Older drugs such as carbamazepine,[567] valproate, and phenytoin have analgesic effects but a relatively higher adverse effect liability than newer agents. Among the new drugs, lamotrigine has been efficacious in several, but not all, studies of neuropathic pain,[568] but carries a small risk for serious cutaneous hypersensitivity, and slow titration is required to reduce this risk. Oxcarbazepine, a metabolite of carbamazepine, has a safer pharmacologic profile and limited evidence of analgesic efficacy,[569] and there is equivocal support for topiramate.[570] Lacosamide, a sodium channel modulator, also yielded analgesic effects in one trial and may be considered if other drugs are not effective.[571] Finally, clonazepam, a benzodiazepine, is favored by some clinicians despite limited supporting data, presumably because its anxiolytic effects are positive.[572]

### Other Drugs Used for Neuropathic Pain

Systemic sodium channel blockers, including intravenous lidocaine and oral antiarrhythmic drugs such as mexiletine, are analgesic.[573,574] A brief intravenous infusion of lidocaine, typically 2 mg/kg to 4 mg/kg infused over 20 to 30 minutes in a monitored setting, can be a useful test for efficacy when prompt relief is needed for neuropathic pain and an opioid is not adequate. Oral mexiletine is rarely tried but is an option for refractory pain.[575]

There is some evidence that one of the commercially available NMDA receptor antagonists, ketamine, has analgesic properties.[576] Ketamine, a dissociative anesthetic, can provide analgesia when infused intravenously or subcutaneously at subanesthetic dosages (eg, 0.1 mg/kg-1.5 mg/kg per hour) or administered orally.[577] The side effect profile, which includes psychotomimetic effects and delirium, may be problematic, however, and the most common use is for short-term therapy in a monitored setting or for refractory terminal pain. Oral NMDA receptor antagonists such as memantine, amantadine, and dextromethorphan have less evidence in support of analgesic effects in neuropathic pain[576,578] and are rarely considered.

Drugs that interact directly with the GABA receptors comprise the $GABA_A$ agonists, specifically the benzodiazepines, and the $GABA_B$ agonists, which include baclofen. The only benzodiazepine generally used for neuropathic pain is clonazepam. Baclofen, an antispasticity drug, improves trigeminal neuralgia and anecdotally is effective for neuropathic pain of other types, including cancer pain.[579] A low starting dose of 5 mg twice daily is gradually titrated to doses that may exceed 200 mg per day for some patients.

### *Drugs Used for Bone Pain*
### Nonsteroidal Antiinflammatory Drugs

Patients with cancer who have multifocal bone pain are usually given an opioid but may benefit with the addition of an NSAID as an adjuvant analgesic used specifically for bone pain. Single-dose NSAID studies demonstrate that this drug class has greater analgesic efficacy than placebo, with an equivalence to 5 mg to 10 mg of intramuscular morphine. Pain scores differ insignificantly for aspirin versus other NSAIDs. Analgesic responses to NSAIDs suggest a weak dose-response relationship.[580] Common side effects include upper GI symptoms, dizziness, and drowsiness. The incidence of side effects tends to increase with dose and time. Single or multiple doses of weak opioids alone or in combination with nonopioid analgesics do not produce greater analgesia than NSAIDs alone. Single doses of weak opioids plus NSAID analgesics produce more side effects than NSAIDs alone.[502,581] However, parecoxib improves morphine responses.[582] Ibuprofen improves oxycodone-acetaminophen responses,[583] and ketorolac adds to the analgesia of parenteral diamorphine.[584]

### Osteoclast Inhibitors

The osteoclast inhibitors (bisphosphonates or denosumab) and bone-seeking radionuclides appear to be better at preventing bone pain than treating established cancer-related bone pain.[585] Bisphosphonates prevent skeletal-related events, including fracture, and substantial data support their analgesic potential.[169,586] This applies to all of the parenteral bisphosphonates including pamidronate, zoledronic acid, ibandronate, and clodronate (not available in the United States). A drug typically is chosen on the basis of experience, cost, and convenience. Standard dosages for pamidronate are 90 mg intravenously on a monthly basis, and for zoledronic acid, 4 mg intravenously monthly. Dose reductions should be made for renal impairment.

The bisphosphonates generally are well-tolerated. A transitory flu-like illness with a pain flare may be reported. The risk of nephrotoxicity, which usually is temporary, necessitates a check of renal function before treatment; if impaired, the starting dose should be lowered and the patient carefully monitored. Although bisphosphonate drugs are used to treat hypercalcemia, the development of symptomatic hypocalcemia following treatment is uncommon in normocalcemic patients who receive the drug for pain. Nonetheless, calcium levels should be monitored during therapy.

There are two other unusual but serious complications associated with the bisphosphonates: osteonecrosis of the jaw[587] and femur fracture.[588] These complications usually occur after months of treatment. Because oral trauma and dental infections increase risk for jaw osteonecrosis, patients with poor dentition should be considered to have a relative contraindication to this therapy.[589]

Denosumab blocks the interaction of RANK ligand to RANK. Standard doses of denosumab are 120 mg subcutaneously every 4 weeks. Denosumab has been found to reduce skeletal-related events better than zoledronic acid.[590] In addition, denosumab appears to delay the onset to malignant-related hypercalcemia better than zoledronic acid, and fewer patients develop hypercalcemia.[591] Denosumab also has been used as an adjuvant in early breast cancer patients receiving aromatase inhibitors. Denosumab reduces the risk of osteoporotic compression fractures,[592] which can occur with hormone deprivation therapy. For relief of established metastatic bone pain, radioisotopes such as Rhenium 223 are better than bisphosphonates and denosumab.[593] Long-term adverse effects of denosumab include osteonecrosis of the jaw (1.9%), which is about the same as with zoledronic acid (1.2%). The incidence of hypocalcemia ranges between 3% and 4%.[594] Risk factors for hypocalcemia include vitamin D deficiency and large tumor burden.[595]

Calcitonin is another osteoclast inhibitor with potential analgesic effects in bone pain. Small controlled trials have yielded conflicting results,[596] however, and this drug is only considered when a bisphosphonate cannot be given. Calcitonin and bisphosphonates are particularly effective for complex regional pain syndrome type 1 pain.[597-599]

### Bone-Seeking Radionuclides

Bone-seeking radionuclides such as strontium-89, rhenium-188 hydroxyethylidene diphosphonate, and samarium-153 link a short-lived radiation source to a bisphosphonate molecule. These compounds can be a useful treatment for multifocal bone pain.[64,600,601] With rhenium-223, relief is experienced by 74% of patients, with a mean duration of 7 weeks and a mean starting time to analgesia of 4 days.[601] Some will have complete pain relief in 1 to 6 months, but there is no evidence that one isotope or dose is superior to another.[602] Myelosuppression is the most significant concern, and treatment requires special skills and facilities. If available, treatment with a bone-seeking radionuclide typically is considered for patients with refractory multifocal bone pain whose blood counts are adequate and who are not expected to require myelosuppressive chemotherapy in the near future.

### Drugs Used for the Pain of Bowel Obstruction

Patients with advanced intraabdominal or pelvic tumors may develop inoperable bowel obstruction associated with pain and other symptoms (see *UNIPAC 4*). Patients whose conditions cannot be managed by stenting[603] or tube decompression potentially can experience good symptom control with medical management.[604] The approach relies on hydration and opioid therapy combined with adjuvant analgesics that address pain, intraluminal secretions, and peristalsis. Useful adjuvant drugs include a corticosteroid,[605,606] anticholinergic agents such as scopolamine or glycopyrrolate, and octreotide.

### Anticholinergic Drugs

Scopolamine can be administered via a transdermal system or parenteral infusion. In the United States, only the hydrobromide salt is available, which crosses the blood-brain barrier and may produce somnolence and confusion. Glycopyrrolate is an anticholinergic drug that has limited ability to cross the blood-brain barrier.[607] It is generally longer acting and has greater antisecretory effects and less cardiac effects. A trial of this drug is preferred when retained alertness is a goal of therapy.

Octreotide, a somatostatin analog, inhibits gastric, pancreatic, and intestinal secretions and reduces gut motility.[608] Small randomized trials demonstrate its efficacy in relieving the symptoms of malignant bowel obstruction.[609-611] The usual starting dose is 100 mcg twice daily, which may be followed by rapid dose titration.[612] Dosages higher than 600 mcg per day rarely are needed. Side effects rarely are a problem, although cost may be a significant issue.

## Nonpharmacological Analgesic Approaches

Although the evidence in support of most nonpharmacological approaches to pain control is limited, these strategies may be valuable in selected patients.[613] They comprise a diverse group of noninvasive and invasive therapies (see Table 6). Most are considered adjunctive to a systemic, opioid-based drug regimen.

### Interventional Approaches

Interventional approaches comprise a large and varied group of injections, neural blockade approaches, and implant therapies.[308,614] The simplest are muscle trigger point and joint injections and local anesthetic infiltration of painful scars.

Neural blockade can be accomplished with local anesthetic (delivered as a bolus or as a perineural infusion) or any of several neurolytic approaches (including chemical neurolysis with alcohol or phenol or mechanical neurolysis using heat or cold).[130] In the past, neurolysis was considered for patients with regional pain in the setting of advanced illness and short life expectancy. The advent of nondestructive approaches such as neuraxial analgesia has largely supplanted this therapy. At present, only celiac plexus block is commonly performed in medically ill populations. This block can effectively address pain from injury to rostral retroperitoneal structures, such as that caused by pancreatic cancer, and may produce fewer side effects than medications.[615] It may be accomplished using any of a variety of percutaneous needle techniques or via an endoscopic ultrasound-guided approach. Referral to an appropriately trained interventional pain specialist, interventional radiologist, or gastroenterologist[616] usually is necessary.

### Other Approaches

Numerous other strategies can be categorized as psychological, rehabilitative, or integrative. Among the most accepted are the mind-body approaches, which are categorized as both psychological and integrative interventions. These treatments should be considered mainstream and are highly useful to address pain and anxiety, enhance coping, and increase self-efficacy.[617] Included among these therapies are interventions that might be encouraged by front-line clinicians, such as relaxation training and guided imagery, and interventions that typically require referral to a trained therapist, such as hypnosis and biofeedback. Relaxation therapy trains patients in a relaxation response induced by repetitive focus on a word, sound, phrase, or body sensation. Guided imagery trains patients to recall specific sights, smells, sounds, tastes, or somatic sensations to engender a positive cognitive and emotional state. These strategies can lessen pain[618,619] and confirm the importance of cognitions and emotions as mediators of symptom distress.

Creative art therapies provide another avenue to realize these benefits. These therapies include music,[620] art, and dance[621] and are usually implemented by trained practitioners who become members of the treatment team. These therapies can provide another means to reduce pain while improving coping and adaptation.

Physical modalities are categorized under rehabilitative strategies. Physical modalities comprise the clinical use of heat or cold, electricity, vibration, or ultrasound. They range from the use of ice packs or heating pads to transcutaneous electrical nerve stimulation to deep muscle ultrasound.[622] Focal musculoskeletal pain is the usual target for these treatments.

Integrative or integrated medicine incorporating complementary or alternative medicine therapies comprise a diverse group of strategies that vary in supporting evidence, familiarity, and use. As noted, the mind-body therapies are mainstream and supported by substantial evidence. Other commonly used approaches in medically ill patients include acupuncture, therapeutic massage, and therapies that incorporate physical movement such as tai chi. Energy approaches (as defined by the National Institutes of Health National Center for Complementary and Alternative Medicine) such as therapeutic touch are also frequently tried despite minimal evidence of efficacy. Trials of biological substances, often suggested from the perspective of a different system such as traditional Chinese medicine, usually are discouraged because of concerns about unanticipated toxicity in the setting of medical illness and the potential for drug-drug interactions. Regardless of the existence of scientific evidence, the use of these approaches is widespread in the United States, and clinicians should carefully ask patients about their use.

## Management of Procedure-Related Pain

Pain associated with diagnostic and therapeutic procedures may contribute greatly to patient suffering and should be controlled. Specific methods to relieve procedure-related pain are available and should be tailored to the procedure itself.[205] Patient education and sensory preparation, amnestic agents, and analgesic interventions are combined for the best result.[623] It is especially important to control procedure-related pain for children[624] (see UNIPAC 8).

Conscious sedation is useful for painful invasive procedures, especially for children. Policies and credentialing are regulated by each healthcare institution. Procedural pain is brief and acute, with little or no time for gradual titration. Become familiar with the administration of opioids and benzodiazepines before attempting to use them to manage procedural pain.[625] Ensure adequate monitoring by skilled personnel other than the person performing the procedure. A healthcare professional skilled in airway management should be present when opioids or sedatives are used for conscious sedation.

## Management of Acute Pain Crises

Episodes of acute pain that occur superimposed on a background of otherwise well-managed chronic pain may represent a flare of an underlying painful condition or a new complication and may require urgent intervention. When pain is very severe it should be considered an urgent situation that often requires admission to a hospital bed.

Specific strategies may be considered to address very severe pain. The first approach usually involves rapid opioid titration, either using repeated boluses or a loading infusion approach. Both approaches are best accomplished using a short-acting drug such as morphine, and careful monitoring is required.

Other pharmacologic approaches may be considered. Administration of a corticosteroid at a high dose, such as dexamethasone, 10 mg intravenously, may be considered for emergent pain that may be associated with inflammation or edema.

Other nonopioid analgesic drugs can be administered by intravenous bolus, including acetaminophen and the NSAIDs ibuprofen or ketorolac. Repeated intravenous lidocaine boluses also may be considered for neuropathic pain starting at 0.5 mg/kg over 30 minutes. The dose can be doubled and then doubled again at intervals of several hours. Severe neuropathic pain also might be addressed through loading boluses of anticonvulsant drugs[626] with potential analgesic effects, such as gabapentin and pregabalin.

Intravenous ketamine infusion also has gained acceptance as an approach to address emerging severe pain.[627] In a monitoring setting, treatment can begin with a small loading bolus and then infused at a low subanesthethic dose, which is again increased every few hours as needed. If available, interventional therapies, such as placement of an epidural or intrathecal catheter for infusion of a local anesthetic and opioid, represent additional options to address uncontrolled severe pain.[628]

Finally, when life expectancy is short, severe pain that cannot quickly be controlled in some other way may be the rationale for a discussion about the role of palliative sedation. Recognizing the indications for this therapy, understanding and communicating its medical and ethical basis, and implementing it appropriately are among the skills that specialists in palliative care can bring to a situation that may be generating high distress for patients, families, and the staff members providing care.[629] (See *UNIPAC 6* and the American Academy of Hospice and Palliative Medicine position statement on palliative sedation, available at aahpm.org/positions/palliative-sedation.

## Clinical Situation

### Joan

Joan is a 66-year-old woman with hepatocellular carcinoma at home with hospice. She is currently on morphine extended release, 60 mg every 12 hours, with morphine elixir, 20 mg every 3 hours as needed, for pain. She describes her pain as mostly right upper quadrant pain that is constant and increases when she takes a deep breath. It is dull in nature but with occasional sharp shooting episodes during the day. She is able to ambulate with assistance at home, eat a small amount, and interact with her family. The nurse calls you and reports that Joan is complaining of more right upper quadrant pain that is not relieved with breakthrough medication. She has doubled her breakthrough morphine with little pain relief and resultant somnolence. She asks if there is anything else we can offer for pain.

 What adjuvant pain medications would you consider for Joan?

Dexamethasone would likely be the best initial choice for liver capsule pain. It also may help associated symptoms such as nausea, anorexia, and depression for patients with advanced disease. Gabapentin is an anticonvulsant medication that is a helpful adjuvant for neuropathic pain. It may take several weeks, however, to titrate up to an effective dose.

### The Case Continues

Joan starts taking scheduled dexamethasone with good results. She has more energy, her appetite increases, and her pain improves for a week. One day, the nurse calls you to report that Joan is sleeping more, eating less, becoming more jaundiced, and is now essentially bedbound. She is grimacing and moving around uncomfortably in bed. The nurse is concerned about the patient not being able to take her extended-release morphine.

 What would you recommend to the hospice nurse?

When patients can no longer take medication by mouth, an alternative route is usually necessary. Options may include a subcutaneous PCA with the equivalent dose of continuous subcutaneous morphine in the place of morphine extended release. A fentanyl patch is not a good option because it has a slow onset of action for this urgent situation and its clearance is delayed with advanced liver disease.

Substituting another long-acting medication via a different route is often considered, but in this rapidly changing situation with progressive liver failure and uncontrolled pain, an immediate-release potent opioid would be the best approach with some frequent doses. The pharmacokinetics of hydromorphone and morphine are relatively stable in liver disease, so either of these two opioids would be reasonable choices.

## The Case Continues

Joan is started on morphine via a subcutaneous PCA, and her pain is well-controlled. She is resting comfortably and occasionally wakes up and says a few words or takes a sip of water, then goes back to sleep. Joan's family is worried that she is oversedated. They express concern that the morphine is hastening her death and feel uncomfortable with the "morphine drip."

 What should be your next response?

Patients with a terminal illness often become less responsive at the end of life. This is a common concern of families at this stage. Because many families do have preconceived ideas about morphine and hastening death, preemptive education about the dying process is important. The best approach is to listen to their concerns and explore the reasons behind them. Families need education about what to expect at the end of life and the role of morphine for comfort.

## The Case Concludes

The physician and nurse make a home visit and talk to the family about what to expect at the end of life and the role of morphine in the subcutaneous route. The family has a better understanding, and they agree to watch closely how a 2 mg/hour morphine infusion rate works. Joan does become more alert but needs more

PCA doses for relief, so the family is convinced the medication is necessary. The family spends quality time with her during her last few days at home, and the infusion rate is adjusted as required. Joan dies comfortably while surrounded by family and friends.

## Patient and Family Education

Patient adherence to a pain management plan improves when healthcare providers take time to listen carefully to the patient's and family's concerns. Concerns about opioid use often are based on common misconceptions. It is important for clinicians to discuss these misconceptions and provide further education about opioids and their treatable side effects. Adherence issues often arise from problems such as swallowing difficulties, concerns about opioid-related constipation, lack of access to expensive medications, and complexity of overall care. Thorough patient and family education is the foundation of effective symptom relief.

# Special Populations

## People with Cancer

Advanced cancer is no longer a terminal illness at diagnosis. Half of patients survive 2 years or more. Persistent pain is an important symptom that increases in prevalence with cancer stage and survival, and that has an impact on patient function (**Table 20**).

Pain occurs in most individuals with advanced cancer. Nearly half of individuals with advanced cancer experience severe pain.[630] In patients with solid tumors, 15% to 75% will experience pain depending on tumor type and stage of cancer.[631] In the case of advanced cancer in which the disease course cannot be modified or in which disease-modifying therapies have been exhausted, guidelines for managing cancer pain was aptly put forth by the European Association for Palliative Care in 2012 and the National Comprehensive Cancer Network in 2016.

Analgesics, mainly opioids, are a mainstay therapy for those with moderate to severe cancer pain. Surveys have shown that opioid therapy for moderate to severe cancer pain reduces pain intensity in a majority of patients.[632] (The same approach to chronic noncancer pain has not been as successful.[633]) However, a multimodal approach (eg, nonpharmacological therapies, surgery, interventional pain treatments/therapies, radiation, cognitive behavioral therapy, neuromodulation, spiritual care) and disease-modifying therapy that targets the underlying cancer illness are more vital additions to analgesic therapy. It takes an interdisciplinary team to best treat cancer pain.

## Analgesic Use for People with Liver Disease

Cirrhosis influences analgesic pharmacokinetics in five major ways: (a) liver cell necrosis resulting in reduced clearance, (b) portal-systemic shunting increasing opioid bioavailability, (c) altered drug-protein binding (affecting albumin more than acid glycoprotein), (d) liver hypoxia, which reduces mixed function oxidase (cytochrome) metabolism more than it does conjugation, and (e) reduced renal function (hepatorenal syndrome).[634] Unlike renal disease, where glomerular filtration rate can be used as a rough guide to adjust doses, there is no reliable marker in liver disease. The Child Pugh Score and Model for End-Stage Liver Disease score are predictors of outcome but are not sensitive to metabolism of individual drugs. The hyperbilirubinemia of biliary obstruction does not cause shunting or reduced cytochrome metabolism relative to a similar bilirubin in end-stage cirrhosis. As a rule, individuals with normal liver synthetic function (normal prothrombin times), normal albumin, absence of ascites, and no history of encephalopathy are unlikely to have altered drug pharmacokinetics.[635]

Taking acetaminophen with liver disease is fraught with hazards. A small proportion of acetaminophen (less than 5%) is metabolized by the cytochrome CYP2EI to N-acetyl-p-benzoquinone imine (NAPQI), which is rendered nontoxic by conjugation to

## Table 20. Cancer-Related Chronic Pain Syndromes[170]

| Related to Tumor | | |
|---|---|---|
| **Mixed Neuropathic/ Nociceptive Syndromes and Nociceptive Syndromes: Somatic** | Tumor-related bone pain | Multifocal bone pain |
| | | Vertebral syndromes |
| | | &bull; Atlanto-axial destruction and odontoid fracture |
| | | &bull; C7-T1 syndrome |
| | | &bull; T12-L1 syndrome |
| | | &bull; Sacral syndrome (back pain secondary to spinal cord compression) |
| | | Pain syndromes related to pelvis and hip |
| | | &bull; Pelvic metastases |
| | | &bull; Hip joint syndrome |
| | | Base of skull metastases |
| | | &bull; Orbital syndrome |
| | | &bull; Parasellar syndrome |
| | | &bull; Middle cranial fossa syndrome |
| | | &bull; Jugular foramen syndrome |
| | | &bull; Occipital condyle syndrome |
| | | &bull; Clivus syndrome |
| | | &bull; Sphenoid sinus syndrome |
| | Tumor-related soft tissue pain | Headache and facial pain |
| | | Ear and eye pain syndromes |
| | | Pleural pain |
| | Paraneoplastic pain syndromes | Muscle cramps |
| | | Other |
| | | &bull; Hypertrophic pulmonary osteoarthropathy |
| | | &bull; Tumor-related gynecomastia |
| | | &bull; Paraneoplastic pemphigus |
| | | &bull; Paraneoplastic Raynaud's phenomenon |

## Table 20. Cancer-Related Chronic Pain Syndromes[170] (continued)

| | |
|---|---|
| **Nociceptive Syndromes: Visceral** | Hepatic distention syndrome |
| | Midline retroperitoneal syndrome |
| | Chronic intestinal obstruction |
| | Peritoneal carcinomatosis |
| | Malignant perineal pain |
| | Adrenal pain syndrome |
| | Ureteric obstruction |
| | |
| **Neuropathic Syndromes** | Leptomeningeal metastases |
| | Painful cranial neuralgias |
| | Glossopharyngeal neuralgia |
| | Trigeminal neuralgia |
| | Malignant painful radiculopathy |
| | Plexopathies |
| |   • Cervical plexopathy |
| |   • Malignant brachial plexopathy |
| |   • Malignant lumbosacral plexopathy |
| |     » Lower lumbosacral plexopathy |
| |     » Sacral plexopathy |
| |     » Panplexopathy |
| |     » Coccygeal plexopathy |
| | Painful peripheral mononeuropathies |
| | Paraneoplastic sensory neuropathy |

Continued on page 108

## Table 20. Cancer-Related Chronic Pain Syndromes[170] (continued)

### Related to Treatment

**Chemotherapy**

Painful peripheral neuropathy, acute and chronic

Raynaud's syndrome

Bony complications of long-term steroids

- Avascular (aseptic) necrosis of femoral or humeral head
- Vertebral compression fractures
- Spinal lipomatosis

**Radiation**

Radiation-induced brachial plexopathy, lumbar plexopathy

Chronic radiation myelopathy

Chronic radiation enteritis and proctitis

Stereotactic radiation induced chest wall pain

Pain secondary to radiation induced lymphedema

Burning perineum syndrome

Osteoradionecrosis

**Surgery**

Postmastectomy pain syndrome

Postradical neck dissection pain

Postthoracotomy pain syndrome

Postthoracotomy frozen shoulder

Postsurgery pelvic floor pain

Stump pain

Phantom pain

*Reprinted from The Lancet, 377(9784), RK Portenoy, Treatment of Cancer Pain, 2236-2247, ©2011, with permission from Elsevier.*

glutathione. The clearance of acetaminophen is delayed in cirrhosis; delayed clearance correlates with prothrombin time and serum albumin.[636,637] However, although the clearance of acetaminophen is delayed, CYP2EI is not increased, and glutathione stores are generally normal.[638] Short-term use and one-time dosing up to 4 g per day appear to be safe; *short-term* in this setting is defined as up to 14 days.[638-640] The American Liver Foundation recommends that individuals with cirrhosis not receive more than 3 g per day. FDA guidelines suggest that for long-term use (more than 14 days) in individuals with cirrhosis, no more than 2 g to 3 g per day should be prescribed.[641] If individuals are actively drinking alcohol or also suffering from malnutrition or cachexia, acetaminophen should not be used.

NSAIDs are largely metabolized by cytochromes and are protein bound, so the clearance of this class of medication will be delayed in advanced cirrhosis. Secondly, the portal-systemic shunt of cirrhosis increases the renin-angiotensin-aldosterone system. Persistent sodium retention plays a role in sustained ascites. The renal response to activation of the renin-angiotensin aldosterone system is to produce vasodilating prostaglandins. Cyclooxygenase inhibitors (COX-1) will counter this compensatory response, resulting in increased ascites and renal failure. Selective cyclooxygenase-2 (COX-2) inhibitors have been used for patients with ascites. In the short term (less than 3 days), there was no renal impairment.[642] However, there is constitutional expression of COX-2 in kidneys, which may be necessary for renal blood flow.[643] In general, both COX-1 and COX-2 inhibitors should be avoided in patients with cirrhosis.

Opioid pharmacokinetics are variably influenced by liver disease depending on the degree of first-pass clearance, whether the particular opioid is metabolized by cytochromes or is conjugated, the type and degree of protein binding, and whether the particular opioid or active metabolites are cleared by the kidneys. Both morphine and hydromorphone have increased bioavailability and prolonged half-life (related to ascites and edema) and delayed clearance.[256,644,645]

Codeine and tramadol must be converted by CYP2D6 to active metabolites for analgesia. Slow clearance of codeine can cause respiratory depression. Hydrocodone and oxycodone are metabolized by CYP2D6 and CYP3A4; both are reduced in advanced cirrhosis.[256,646,647] There can be a marked delay in clearance of oxycodone.[648] Methadone and fentanyl are also metabolized by cytochromes CYP2B6 and CYP3A4, respectively, which are reduced in advanced liver disease. Fentanyl is also bound to albumin.[634] Buprenorphine is metabolized to the weakly active metabolite norbuprenorphine by CYP3A4, but both the parent opioid and metabolite are glucuronidated, which is rate-limiting. Glucuronidation, unlike cytochromes, is relatively well-preserved in liver disease. Chronic liver disease results in increased uridine 5'-diphosphate-glucuronosyltransferase in remaining viable hepatocytes.[649-651] Both the parent drug, buprenorphine, and metabolite are eliminated in feces and are independent of renal function. For this reason, buprenorphine is a safer drug than fentanyl to use in advanced liver disease.[651]

Several important prescribing recommendations should be considered. For those with advanced liver disease (ascites, increased prothrombin time, low albumin, history of encephalopathy), opioid doses should be 50% or less of those used when liver function is normal, without cirrhosis. Transdermal fentanyl and sustained-release potent opioids should not be used. Individuals should be started on immediate-release potent opioids. Conjugated opioids (eg, hydromorphone, morphine, buprenorphine, levorphanol) may be preferred over opioids requiring cytochrome metabolism for clearance. For those with hepatorenal failure, buprenorphine may be preferred over morphine and hydromorphone. Patients should be educated about opioid side effects and have telephone access to case managers, nurses, or prescribing physicians. Benzodiazepines, sedatives, and hypnotics as well as anticholinergics should be avoided. Adjuvant analgesics should be used cautiously and not added when initially starting opioids. Gabapentinoids are safe because this class of drug is not metabolized by the liver. However, doses will have to be adjusted if renal function declines.

## Children

When assessing pain in children, careful attention should be paid to the following issues:

- the child's developmental stage and its effect on the meanings of pain and the understanding of the child's prognosis
- the child-parent relationship
- underreporting of pain by parents when compared with the child's self-report
- the common occurrence of regression, such as an increase in dependence behaviors during profound illness
- medication doses based on weight (ie, mg/kg/dose)
- individualized assessment and monitoring (there is no "standard dose" for a child).

Nonverbal assessments of pain (eg, crying, grimace, heart rate) are important in the pediatric patient population. When considering assessments of pain, the developmental stage of the child is critical. For example, a 4-year-old child should be able to use a 4-point scale (eg, poker chip tool). Be sure to use terminology the child understands (eg, "ow," "boo boo"). A 7-year-old has increased vocabulary and should be able to use a 10-point Likert scale.

The high-dose chemotherapy agents used to treat cancer in children often result in treatment-related conditions such as neuropathies, mouth ulcers, and joint pain that may cause more pain than the disease itself, particularly in the case of leukemia.[652] When caring for children, adequately assessing and managing treatment-related sources of pain often is as important as adequately controlling cancer-related pain[653] (see UNIPAC 7).

Start with the recommended dosage and rapidly titrate to effect; this often results in a final dosage several times higher than the starting dosage. For children younger than 6 months, start at lower dosages because young infants have less mature liver and kidney function and different ratios of water to fat influencing bioavailability. (For recommended initial opioid dosages for children and more information on pediatric pain management, see UNIPAC 7.)

## Older Adults

Older patients tend to prefer categorical scales over visual analogue scales for pain severity. However, the use of a visual analogue scale, numerical scale, or categorical scale can be used with equal efficacy.[654] Given the number of older, nonverbal patients who struggle with self-reporting their pain, it is critical to also assess and document nonverbal signs of pain. If nonverbal signs of pain are present (eg, grimace, restlessness, agitation), a time-limited trial of individualized analgesics targeting likely etiologies is critical.

### Pain, Analgesia, and Older Individuals

One retrospective study of three groups of patients—those younger than 65 years, those aged 65 to 74 years, and those older than 75 years—evaluated trajectory of symptoms during the course of illness. Interestingly, there was no difference in the trajectory of symptoms between the three age groups. Near the end of life, pain and nausea diminished among all groups.[655] The use of various symptom-related medications, except opioids, diminished over time in all groups. There was no difference in pain intensity between the younger group and older group; however, there were differences in dosages of opioids being used, which were lower in the older group.[656]

Moderate or more severe pain has been shown to be independently associated with frailty.[657] In addition, a lower prevalence of breakthrough pain and fewer opioid rotations have been reported for the older population.[658] Similar findings in older patients have been previously published.[659-662] In general, there is a lack of association between pain intensity and opioid consumption in the older population. The physiological decline in renal function that occurs with aging may account for the reduced need for opioids at the end of life.[663] Due to sarcopenia associated with aging and comorbid cachexia, the serum creatinine may be in the "normal" range for older adults and not reflect renal function. Physicians often miss renal dysfunction in older people.[664]

Older adults have a 10% to 25% increased risk of developing adverse effects from opioids relative to younger patients.[665] The adverse cognitive effects experienced by older people are related to underlying comorbidities, polypharmacy, and reduced tolerance to adverse drug effects.[663] Many clinicians are hesitant to prescribe opioids for this population because they fear precipitating side effects such as delirium, sedation, constipation, and falls. Despite older people's increased susceptibility to adverse drug reactions, analgesic medications, including opioids, can be used successfully with this population.[666] It is particularly helpful to counsel older patients and their family members about the safety and potential side effects of opioids. Physicians should reassure patients and family members that these side effects are not universal and can be avoided or treated if necessary.[667]

Particular effort to review potentially inappropriate medication use in older adults (ie, Beers Criteria) and drug-drug interactions is essential in this patient population.[668] Close monitoring is critical, given that many drugs depend on renal clearance.[669] In frail, older patients, drugs should be started at low dosages (eg, half the standard adult dosage), such as

2.5 mg of oxycodone. Frequent monitoring should enable careful dose titration if pain is not under control. Side effects should be anticipated and managed preventively when appropriate. Drugs with lesser effects on the CNS, such as nonopioid analgesics or topical agents, should be considered for coanalgesic therapy. Nonpharmacologic strategies also should be used when possible. The addition of these agents and strategies may reduce the overall amount of opioid needed to control a patient's pain.[670] When confusion arises for older patients who are undergoing opioid therapy, look for reversible causes such as urinary or fecal retention, urinary tract infection, or metabolic or electrolyte abnormalities and reduce CNS-active medications before considering an opioid switch or rotation.[671] If an opioid rotation is being considered, the physician should be aware of potential drug-drug and drug-disease interactions that may occur with the newly prescribed opioid. For instance, many older individuals have cardiovascular disease and may have a prolonged QTc interval on the electrocardiogram.[671] Methadone would be a less safe option for this group of patients. On the other hand, if the patient has reduced renal function and no evidence of risk factors for a prolonged QTc interval, low-dose methadone may be a reasonable option.

### Particular Opioid Choices for Older Individuals
Unfortunately there are no randomized trials of opioid use by older patients. A retrospective chart review was conducted for 10 carefully selected older patients with a mean age of 76 years. The starting dose of morphine for all patients was 1 mg to 3 mg three times per day, and maintenance dosages ranged from 5 mg to 30 mg per day. Pain improved significantly overall and was maintained for 14 months (range, 10-21 months).[672] In two open-label trials of transdermal buprenorphine, a subset of older patients tolerated opioid therapy well without increased adverse effects.[347,673] In a study from China, transdermal fentanyl was determined to be safe for people between the ages of 60 and 90 years (mean age, 71 years).[674] From a pooled analysis of three randomized trials, extended-release tapentadol appeared to be safe and effective for those older than 75 years.[675] Finally, in a group of patients older than 70 years, oxycodone-naloxone prolonged release was effective in treating noncancer pain for a prolonged period of time but at low dosages (less than 20 mg of oxycodone per day).[676]

A consensus panel of experts reviewed the published literature in 2008.[677] The panel recommended buprenorphine for several reasons. Buprenorphine transdermal is convenient because it comes as a 7-day patch. Because buprenorphine has antihyperalgesia characteristics, it is effective with neuropathic pain commonly experienced by older individuals.[677] All opioids except buprenorphine have prolonged clearance of the parent opioid and metabolites in older patients and those with reduced renal function. Reasons for using buprenorphine put forth by multiple investigators include less constipation, reduced risk for falls, and reduced hypogonadism relative to other potent opioids.[404,421,678,679]

### Adjuvant Analgesics in Older Individuals
The Beers list of medications should be consulted when choosing adjuvant analgesics for older patients. Adjuvant analgesics commonly are used when treating pain experienced by older

patients.[680] Adjuvant analgesics may be "opioid sparing," which could limit opioid toxicity. However, two studies suggest that adjuvant analgesics do not reduce opioid doses or prevent opioid rotation.[681,682] Acetaminophen is preferred over NSAIDs.[683] Acetaminophen doses should be limited to 3 g daily for older patients. Secondary amine tricyclic antidepressants, nortriptyline, and desipramine are preferred over amitriptyline because amine antidepressants are less anticholinergic.[663] The evidence for effective pain control using desipramine is not as well-established as for amitriptyline.[529] SSRIs lack anticholinergic activity but come with little evidence to support their use as an adjuvant analgesic.[684] SSRIs not only block cytochromes but also can interact with tramadol, oxycodone, methadone, and fentanyl, leading to serotonin syndrome and delirium.[685-687] Duloxetine and venlafaxine have a wider therapeutic index than tricyclic antidepressants. Duloxetine is well-tolerated by older patients.[688,689] Treatment-emergent adverse events for duloxetine include dry mouth, constipation, nausea, diarrhea, dizziness, and fatigue. Gabapentinoids are better tolerated, but both gabapentin and pregabalin are subject to renal clearance and can cause edema, sedation, and cognitive dysfunction. Gabapentin is the most commonly prescribed drug, with a frequency of 29%, and it is used mainly for anxiety disorders, psychosis, neuropathic pain, and mood disorders.[690]

## People with Advanced Dementia

Assessing pain can be challenging with patients who have advanced dementia. These patients may have difficulty communicating when experiencing pain. It should be assumed that these patients experience pain, although their ability to process and respond to it often is altered. Instead, they may respond to a noxious stimulus by exhibiting a sudden change in behavior such as physical aggressiveness or social withdrawal.[691,692]

Some patients with advanced dementia can self-report, and it is important to always ask if they are feeling pain. Caregivers and family members who know the patient well also can be queried. With nonverbal patients, behavioral indicators such as facial expressions, body movements, vocalizations, and changes in interpersonal interactions or activity patterns may serve as essential data to assess pain.[691] Several validated assessment tools are available for use with patients who have advanced dementia. The Assessment of Discomfort in Dementia protocol,[693] Discomfort Scale for Dementia of the Alzheimer's Type,[694] Pain Assessment in Advanced Dementia scale,[695] and Checklist of Nonverbal Pain Indicators[696] are several examples (see *UNIPAC 9*).

## People from Diverse Cultures

Analgesic treatment disparities among various cultures are gaining more attention.[697,698] For example, studies of opioid treatment disparities for African Americans remain consistent across pain types, settings, study quality, and data collection periods.[699] The size of the difference is sufficiently large to raise not only normative but also quality and safety concerns.[699] The literature suggests that the sources of pain disparities among racial and ethnic minorities are complex, involving patient (eg, patient/healthcare provider communication, attitudes), healthcare provider (eg, decision making), and healthcare system (eg, access to pain medication) factors.[700]

When assessing pain experienced by patients from diverse cultures, careful attention should be paid to the following issues:

- cultural differences in the meanings of pain[701,702]
- cultural differences in religious practices[703]
- cultural expectations regarding reactions to pain, such as stoicism or emotional expression[698,704]
- cultural differences in how information is shared and expressed
- communication barriers with patients who speak a different language
- mistrust of the medical system based on historical or personal experiences.[705]

# Future Outlook for Pain Management

There are reasons to hope for better pain management in the future as research continues and medical evidence accumulates. New pharmacological and nonpharmacological treatments for pain will become available. Standardized measures of clinical outcomes in pain management are being developed that will allow further development of standards of care.

Palliative care specialists are at the forefront of advocacy for the dignity and humane treatment of those with serious life-limiting illnesses and their families. Relieving pain and suffering, regardless of its source, is congruent with our ethic and essential to our task.

# References

1.  Boland E, Eiser C, Ezaydi Y, Greenfield DM, Ahmedzai SH, Snowden JA. Living with advanced but stable multiple myeloma: a study of the symptom burden and cumulative effects of disease and intensive (hematopoietic stem cell transplant-based) treatment on health-related quality of life. *J Pain Symptom Manage*. 2013;46(5):671-680.

2.  Lee TH. Zero pain is not the goal. *JAMA*. 2016;315(15):1575-1577.

3.  Mularski RA, White-Chu F, Overbay D, Miller L, Asch SM, Ganzini L. Measuring pain as the 5th vital sign does not improve quality of pain management. *J Gen Intern Med*. 2006;21(6):607-612.

4.  Zubkoff L, Lorenz KA, Lanto AB, et al. Does screening for pain correspond to high quality care for veterans? *J Gen Intern Med*. 2010;25(9):900-905.

5.  Paulozzi LJ, Weisler RH, Patkar AA. A national epidemic of unintentional prescription opioid overdose deaths: how physicians can help control it. *J Clin Psychiatry*. 2011;72(5):589-592.

6.  Scherrer JF, Salas J, Copeland LA, et al. Increased risk of depression recurrence after initiation of prescription opioids in noncancer pain patients. *J Pain*. 2016;17(4):473-482.

7.  Scherrer JF, Salas J, Bucholz KK, et al. New depression diagnosis following prescription of codeine, hydrocodone or oxycodone. *Pharmacoepidemiol Drug Saf*. 2016;25(5):560-568.

8.  Scherrer JF, Salas J, Copeland LA, et al. Prescription opioid duration, dose, and increased risk of depression in 3 large patient populations. *Ann Fam Med*. 2016;14(1):54-62.

9.  Kolodny A, Courtwright DT, Hwang CS, et al. The prescription opioid and heroin crisis: a public health approach to an epidemic of addiction. *Annu Rev Public Health*. 2015;36:559-574.

10. Ballantyne JC, Sullivan MD. Intensity of chronic pain—the wrong metric? *N Engl J Med*. 2015;373(22):2098-2099.

11. Chen L, Vo T, Seefeld L, et al. Lack of correlation between opioid dose adjustment and pain score change in a group of chronic pain patients. *J Pain*. 2013;14(4):384-392.

12. Serlin RC, Mendoza TR, Nakamura Y, Edwards KR, Cleeland CS. When is cancer pain mild, moderate or severe? Grading pain severity by its interference with function. *Pain*. 1995;61(2):277-284.

13. Sullivan MD, Ballantyne JC. Must we reduce pain intensity to treat chronic pain? *Pain*. 2016;157(1):65-69.

14. Campbell JN. The fifth vital sign revisited. *Pain*. 2016;157(1):3-4.

15. Morone NE, Weiner DK. Pain as the fifth vital sign: exposing the vital need for pain education. *Clin Ther*. 2013;35(11):1728-1732.

16. Cassell EJ. The nature of suffering and the goals of medicine. *N Engl J Med*. 1982;306(11):639-645.

17. Sela RA, Bruera E, Conner-Spady B, Cumming C, Walker C. Sensory and affective dimensions of advanced cancer pain. *Psychooncology*. 2002;11(1):23-34.

18. Zaza C, Baine N. Cancer pain and psychosocial factors: a critical review of the literature. *J Pain Symptom Manage*. 2002;24(5):526-542.

19. Coyle N. The existential slap—a crisis of disclosure. *Int J Palliat Nurs*. 2004;10(11):520.

20. Ong CK, Forbes D. Embracing Cicely Saunders's concept of total pain. *BMJ*. 2005;331(7516):576.

21. Saunders C. Drug treatment in the terminal stages of cancer. *Curr Med Drugs*. 1960;1(1):16-28.

22. Saunders C. Care of the dying 3: control of pain in terminal cancer. *Nurs Times*. October 23 1959:1031-1032.

23. Saunders C. *The Management of Terminal Illness*. London, UK: Hospital Medicine Publications Ltd.; 1967.

24. Saunders C. The Moment of Truth: Care of the Dying Person. In: Pearson L, ed. *Death and Dying: Current Issues in the Treatment of the Dying Person*. Cleveland, OH: The Press of Case Western Reserve University; 1969:49-78.

25. Saunders C. An Individual Approach to the Relief of Pain. *People and Cancer.* London: The British Council; 1970:34-38.

26. Saunders C. Current views on pain relief and terminal care. In: Swerdlow M, ed. *The Therapy of Pain.* Lancaster: MTP Press; 1981.

27. Dowell D, Haegerich TM, Chou R. CDC guideline for prescribing opioids for chronic pain—United States, 2016. *JAMA.* 2016;315(15):1624-1645.

28. Dahlin CM, Kelley JM, Jackson VA, Temel JS. Early palliative care for lung cancer: improving quality of life and increasing survival. *Int J Palliat Nurs.* 2010;16(9):420-423.

29. Temel JS, Greer JA, Muzikansky A, et al. Early palliative care for patients with metastatic non-small-cell lung cancer. *N Engl J Med.* 2010;363(8):733-742.

30. Zimmermann C, Swami N, Krzyzanowska M, et al. Early palliative care for patients with advanced cancer: a cluster-randomised controlled trial. *Lancet.* 2014;383(9930):1721-1730.

31. Scherrer JF, Svrakic DM, Freedland KE, et al. Prescription opioid analgesics increase the risk of depression. *J Gen Intern Med.* 2014;29(3):491-499.

32. Scherrer JF, Salas J, Lustman PJ, Burge S, Schneider FD. Change in opioid dose and change in depression in a longitudinal primary care patient cohort. *Pain.* 2015;156(2):348-355.

33. Dale R, Edwards J, Ballantyne J. Opioid risk assessment in palliative medicine. *J Community Support Oncol.* 2016;14(3):94-100.

34. Gregorian RS, Jr., Gasik A, Kwong WJ, Voeller S, Kavanagh S. Importance of side effects in opioid treatment: a trade-off analysis with patients and physicians. *J Pain.* 2010;11(11):1095-1108.

35. Boswell K, Kwong WJ, Kavanagh S. Burden of opioid-associated gastrointestinal side effects from clinical and economic perspectives: a systematic literature review. *J Opioid Manag.* 2010;6(4):269-289.

36. Porreca F, Ossipov MH. Nausea and vomiting side effects with opioid analgesics during treatment of chronic pain: mechanisms, implications, and management options. *Pain Med.* 2009;10(4):654-662.

37. Hayhurst CJ, Durieux ME. Differential opioid tolerance and opioid-induced hyperalgesia: a clinical reality. *Anesthesiology.* 2016;124(2):483-488.

38. Bawor M, Bami H, Dennis BB, et al. Testosterone suppression in opioid users: a systematic review and meta-analysis. *Drug Alcohol Depend.* 2015;149:1-9.

39. Daniell HW. Opioid osteoporosis. *Arch Intern Med.* 2004;164(3):338.

40. Ballantyne JC, Sullivan MD. Intensity of chronic pain. *N Engl J Med.* 2016;374(14):1395.

41. Ballantyne JC, Kalso E, Stannard C. WHO analgesic ladder: a good concept gone astray. *BMJ.* 2016;352:i20.

42. Peerdeman KJ, van Laarhoven AI, Keij SM, et al. Relieving patients' pain with expectation interventions: a meta-analysis. *Pain.* 2016.

43. Ballantyne JC. Opioid therapy in chronic pain. *Phys Med Rehabil Clin N Am.* 2015;26(2):201-218.

44. Ballantyne JC. Avoiding opioid analgesics for treatment of chronic low back pain. *JAMA.* 2016;315(22):2459-2460.

45. Cassell EJ. Diagnosing suffering: a perspective. *Ann Intern Med.* 1999;131(7):531-534.

46. Cassell EJ. The nature of suffering: physical, psychological, social, and spiritual aspects. *NLN Publ.* 1992(15-2461):1-10.

47. Cassell EJ. Recognizing suffering. *Hastings Cent Rep.* 1991;21(3):24-31.

48. Cassell EJ. The relief of suffering. *Arch Intern Med.* 1983;143(3):522-523.

49. Edwards RR, Dworkin RH, Turk DC, et al. Patient phenotyping in clinical trials of chronic pain treatments: IMMPACT recommendations. *Pain.* 2016;157(9):1851-1871.

50. van der Leeuw J, Ridker PM, van der Graaf Y, Visseren FL. Personalized cardiovascular disease prevention by applying individualized prediction of treatment effects. *Eur Heart J.* 2014;35(13):837-843.

51. Task Force on Taxonomy of the International Association for the Study of Pain. *Classification of Chronic Pain.* Seattle, WA: IASP Press; 1994.

52. Gallagher RM. Chronification to maldynia: biopsychosocial failure of pain homeostasis. *Pain Med.* 2011;12(7):993-995.

53. Dickinson BD, Head CA, Gitlow S, Osbahr AJ, 3rd. Maldynia: pathophysiology and management of neuropathic and maladaptive pain—a report of the AMA Council on Science and Public Health. *Pain Med.* 2010;11(11):1635-1653.

54. Giordano J. Maldynia: chronic pain as illness, and the need for complementarity in pain care. *Forsch Komplementmed.* 2008;15(5):277-281.

55. Baron R, Binder A, Wasner G. Neuropathic pain: diagnosis, pathophysiological mechanisms, and treatment. *Lancet Neurol.* 2010;9(8):807-819.

56. Bouhassira D, Attal N. Translational neuropathic pain research: a clinical perspective. *Neuroscience.* 2016.

57. Treede RD, Rief W, Barke A, et al. A classification of chronic pain for ICD-11. *Pain.* 2015;156(6):1003-1007.

58. Arthur J, Yennurajalingam S, Nguyen L, et al. The routine use of the Edmonton Classification System for Cancer Pain in an outpatient supportive care center. *Palliat Support Care.* 2015;13(5):1185-1192.

59. Aronoff GM. What do we know about the pathophysiology of chronic pain? Implications for treatment considerations. *Med Clin North Am.* 2016;100(1):31-42.

60. Yarnitsky D. Role of endogenous pain modulation in chronic pain mechanisms and treatment. *Pain.* 2015;156 Suppl 1:S24-31.

61. Nir RR, Yarnitsky D. Conditioned pain modulation. *Curr Opin Support Palliat Care.* 2015;9(2):131-137.

62. Heinricher MM, Tavares I, Leith JL, Lumb BM. Descending control of nociception: specificity, recruitment and plasticity. *Brain Res Rev.* 2009;60(1):214-225.

63. Heinricher MM. Pain modulation and the transition from acute to chronic pain. *Adv Exp Med Biol.* 2016;904:105-115.

64. Institute of Medicine (US) Forum on Neuroscience and Nervous System Disorders. *Sex Differences and Implications for Translational Neuroscience Research: Workshop Summary.* Washington, DC: National Academy of Sciences;2011.

65. Yarnitsky D. Conditioned pain modulation (the diffuse noxious inhibitory control-like effect): its relevance for acute and chronic pain states. *Curr Opin Anaesthesiol.* 2010;23(5):611-615.

66. Nahman-Averbuch H, Yarnitsky D, Granovsky Y, et al. Pronociceptive pain modulation in patients with painful chemotherapy-induced polyneuropathy. *J Pain Symptom Manage.* 2011;42(2):229-238.

67. Yarnitsky D, Granot M, Nahman-Averbuch H, Khamaisi M, Granovsky Y. Conditioned pain modulation predicts duloxetine efficacy in painful diabetic neuropathy. *Pain.* 2012;153(6):1193-1198.

68. Potvin S, Marchand S. Pain facilitation and pain inhibition during conditioned pain modulation in fibromyalgia and in healthy controls. *Pain.* 2016;157(8):1704-1710.

69. Staud R. Abnormal endogenous pain modulation is a shared characteristic of many chronic pain conditions. *Expert Rev Neurother.* 2012;12(5):577-585.

70. Cleary DR, Neubert MJ, Heinricher MM. Are opioid-sensitive neurons in the rostral ventromedial medulla inhibitory interneurons? *Neuroscience.* 2008;151(2):564-571.

71. Barr GA, Wang S. Analgesia induced by localized injection of opiate peptides into the brain of infant rats. *Eur J Pain.* 2013;17(5):676-691.

72. Ossipov MH, Lai J, King T, Vanderah TW, Porreca F. Underlying mechanisms of pronociceptive consequences of prolonged morphine exposure. *Biopolymers.* 2005;80(2-3):319-324.

73. Mase H, Sakai A, Sakamoto A, Suzuki H. A subset of mu-opioid receptor-expressing cells in the rostral ventromedial medulla contribute to thermal hyperalgesia in experimental neuropathic pain. *Neurosci Res.* 2011;70(1):35-43.

74. Vanderah TW, Suenaga NM, Ossipov MH, Malan TP, Jr., Lai J, Porreca F. Tonic descending facilitation from the rostral ventromedial medulla mediates opioid-induced abnormal pain and antinociceptive tolerance. *J Neurosci.* 2001;21(1):279-286.

75. Schepers RJ, Mahoney JL, Shippenberg TS. Inflammation-induced changes in rostral ventromedial medulla mu and kappa opioid receptor mediated antinociception. *Pain.* 2008;136(3):320-330.

76. Kincaid W, Neubert MJ, Xu M, Kim CJ, Heinricher MM. Role for medullary pain facilitating neurons in secondary thermal hyperalgesia. *J Neurophysiol.* 2006;95(1):33-41.

77. Upadhyay J, Maleki N, Potter J, et al. Alterations in brain structure and functional connectivity in prescription opioid-dependent patients. *Brain.* 2010;133(Pt 7):2098-2114.

78. Upadhyay J, Anderson J, Baumgartner R, et al. Modulation of CNS pain circuitry by intravenous and sublingual doses of buprenorphine. *Neuroimage.* 2012;59(4):3762-3773.

79. Upadhyay J, Anderson J, Schwarz AJ, et al. Imaging drugs with and without clinical analgesic efficacy. *Neuropsychopharmacology.* 2011;36(13):2659-2673.

80. Jimenez-Andrade JM, Mantyh WG, Bloom AP, Ferng AS, Geffre CP, Mantyh PW. Bone cancer pain. *Ann N Y Acad Sci.* 2010;1198:173-181.

81. Bennett GJ. Pathophysiology and animal models of cancer-related painful peripheral neuropathy. *Oncologist.* 2010;15 Suppl 2:9-12.

82. Hjermstad MJ, Fainsinger R, Kaasa S. Assessment and classification of cancer pain. *Curr Opin Support Palliat Care.* 2009;3(1):24-30.

83. Lechner B, Chow S, Chow R, et al. The incidence of neuropathic pain in bone metastases patients referred for palliative radiotherapy. *Radiother Oncol.* 2016;118(3):557-561.

84. Karshikoff B, Jensen KB, Kosek E, et al. Why sickness hurts: a central mechanism for pain induced by peripheral inflammation. *Brain Behav Immun.* 2016;57:38-46.

85. Hannestad J, Gallezot JD, Schafbauer T, et al. Endotoxin-induced systemic inflammation activates microglia: [(1)(1)C]PBR28 positron emission tomography in nonhuman primates. *Neuroimage.* 2012;63(1):232-239.

86. Ren K, Dubner R. Interactions between the immune and nervous systems in pain. *Nat Med.* 2010;16(11):1267-1276.

87. DeVon HA, Piano MR, Rosenfeld AG, Hoppensteadt DA. The association of pain with protein inflammatory biomarkers: a review of the literature. *Nurs Res.* 2014;63(1):51-62.

88. Kadetoff D, Lampa J, Westman M, Andersson M, Kosek E. Evidence of central inflammation in fibromyalgia-increased cerebrospinal fluid interleukin-8 levels. *J Neuroimmunol.* 2012;242(1-2):33-38.

89. Mantyh P. Bone cancer pain: causes, consequences, and therapeutic opportunities. *Pain.* 2013;154:S54-S62.

90. American Pain Society. APS Glossary of Pain Terminology. APS Pain Society Website. http://americanpainsociety.org. Accessed September 17, 2007.

91. Caraceni A, Zecca E, Martini C, Pigni A, Bracchi P. Gabapentin for breakthrough pain due to bone metastases. *Palliat Med.* 2008;22(4):392-393.

92. Peters CM, Ghilardi JR, Keyser CP, et al. Tumor-induced injury of primary afferent sensory nerve fibers in bone cancer pain. *Exp Neurol.* 2005;193(1):85-100.

93. Donovan-Rodriguez T, Dickenson AH, Urch CE. Gabapentin normalizes spinal neuronal responses that correlate with behavior in a rat model of cancer-induced bone pain. *Anesthesiology.* 2005;102(1):132-140.

94. Arendt-Nielsen L, Frokjaer JB, Staahl C, et al. Effects of gabapentin on experimental somatic pain and temporal summation. *Reg Anesth Pain Med*. 2007;32(5):382-388.

95. Falk S, Dickenson AH. Pain and nociception: mechanisms of cancer-induced bone pain. *J Clin Oncol*. 2014;32(16):1647-1654.

96. Falk S, Bannister K, Dickenson AH. Cancer pain physiology. *Br J Pain*. 2014;8(4):154-162.

97. Urch C. The pathophysiology of cancer-induced bone pain: current understanding. *Palliat Med*. 2004;18(4):267-274.

98. Drake MT, Clarke BL, Khosla S. Bisphosphonates: mechanism of action and role in clinical practice. *Mayo Clin Proc*. 2008;83(9):1032-1045.

99. Lipton A, Jacobs I. Denosumab: benefits of RANK ligand inhibition in cancer patients. *Curr Opin Support Palliat Care*. 2011;5(3):258-264.

100. Jimenez Andrade JM, Mantyh P. Cancer pain: from the development of mouse models to human clinical trials. In: Kruger L, Light AR, eds. *Translational Pain Research: From Mouse to Man*. Boca Raton, FL: CRC Press/Taylor & Francis; 2010.

101. Mantyh PW. A mechanism-based understanding of bone cancer pain. *Novartis Found Symp*. 2004;261:194-214; discussion 214-199, 256-161.

102. Mantyh PW, Hunt SP. Mechanisms that generate and maintain bone cancer pain. *Novartis Found Symp*. 2004;260:221-238; discussion 238-240, 277-229.

103. Jimenez-Andrade JM, Bloom AP, Stake JI, et al. Pathological sprouting of adult nociceptors in chronic prostate cancer-induced bone pain. *J Neurosci*. 2010;30(44):14649-14656.

104. Mantyh WG, Jimenez-Andrade JM, Stake JI, et al. Blockade of nerve sprouting and neuroma formation markedly attenuates the development of late stage cancer pain. *Neuroscience*. 2010;171(2):588-598.

105. Gould HJ, 3rd, Gould TN, England JD, Paul D, Liu ZP, Levinson SR. A possible role for nerve growth factor in the augmentation of sodium channels in models of chronic pain. *Brain Res*. 2000;854(1-2):19-29.

106. Ji RR, Samad TA, Jin SX, Schmoll R, Woolf CJ. p38 MAPK activation by NGF in primary sensory neurons after inflammation increases TRPV1 levels and maintains heat hyperalgesia. *Neuron*. 2002;36(1):57-68.

107. Brown MT, Herrmann DN, Goldstein M, et al. Nerve safety of tanezumab, a nerve growth factor inhibitor for pain treatment. *J Neurol Sci*. 2014;345(1-2):139-147.

108. Hutchinson MR, Shavit Y, Grace PM, Rice KC, Maier SF, Watkins LR. Exploring the neuroimmunopharmacology of opioids: an integrative review of mechanisms of central immune signaling and their implications for opioid analgesia. *Pharmacol Rev*. 2011;63(3):772-810.

109. Lin SL, Chang FL, Ho SY, Charoenkwan P, Wang KW, Huang HL. Predicting neuroinflammation in morphine tolerance for tolerance therapy from immunostaining images of rat spinal cord. *PLoS One*. 2015;10(10):e0139806.

110. International Association for the Study of Pain. IASP Taxonomy. https://www.iasp-pain.org/Taxonomy. Accessed July 12, 2017.

111. Bennett MI, Rayment C, Hjermstad M, Aass N, Caraceni A, Kaasa S. Prevalence and aetiology of neuropathic pain in cancer patients: a systematic review. *Pain*. 2012;153(2):359-365.

112. Treede RD, Jensen TS, Campbell JN, et al. Neuropathic pain: redefinition and a grading system for clinical and research purposes. *Neurology*. 2008;70(18):1630-1635.

113. Amir R, Kocsis JD, Devor M. Multiple interacting sites of ectopic spike electrogenesis in primary sensory neurons. *J Neurosci*. 2005;25(10):2576-2585.

114. Devor M. Ectopic discharge in Abeta afferents as a source of neuropathic pain. *Exp Brain Res*. 2009;196(1):115-128.

115. Biggs JE, Yates JM, Loescher AR, Clayton NM, Robinson PP, Boissonade FM. Effect of SB-750364, a specific TRPV1 receptor antagonist, on injury-induced ectopic discharge in the lingual nerve. *Neurosci Lett.* 2008;443(1):41-45.

116. Nazemi S, Manaheji H, Noorbakhsh SM, et al. Inhibition of microglial activity alters spinal wide dynamic range neuron discharge and reduces microglial Toll-like receptor 4 expression in neuropathic rats. *Clin Exp Pharmacol Physiol.* 2015;42(7):772-779.

117. Liu FY, Qu XX, Cai J, Wang FT, Xing GG, Wan Y. Electrophysiological properties of spinal wide dynamic range neurons in neuropathic pain rats following spinal nerve ligation. *Neurosci Bull.* 2011;27(1):1-8.

118. Weissner W, Winterson BJ, Stuart-Tilley A, Devor M, Bove GM. Time course of substance P expression in dorsal root ganglia following complete spinal nerve transection. *J Comp Neurol.* 2006;497(1):78-87.

119. Christensen MD, Hulsebosch CE. Spinal cord injury and anti-NGF treatment results in changes in CGRP density and distribution in the dorsal horn in the rat. *Exp Neurol.* 1997;147(2):463-475.

120. Sarantopoulos C, McCallum B, Sapunar D, Kwok WM, Hogan Q. ATP-sensitive potassium channels in rat primary afferent neurons: the effect of neuropathic injury and gabapentin. *Neurosci Lett.* 2003;343(3):185-189.

121. Busserolles J, Tsantoulas C, Eschalier A, Lopez Garcia JA. Potassium channels in neuropathic pain: advances, challenges, and emerging ideas. *Pain.* 2016;157 Suppl 1:S7-14.

122. Hoot MR, Sim-Selley LJ, Selley DE, Scoggins KL, Dewey WL. Chronic neuropathic pain in mice reduces mu-opioid receptor-mediated G-protein activity in the thalamus. *Brain Res.* 2011;1406:1-7.

123. Diamond J, Foerster A, Holmes M, Coughlin M. Sensory nerves in adult rats regenerate and restore sensory function to the skin independently of endogenous NGF. *J Neurosci.* 1992;12(4):1467-1476.

124. Diamond J, Holmes M, Coughlin M. Endogenous NGF and nerve impulses regulate the collateral sprouting of sensory axons in the skin of the adult rat. *J Neurosci.* 1992;12(4):1454-1466.

125. Doubell TP, Mannion RJ, Woolf CJ. Intact sciatic myelinated primary afferent terminals collaterally sprout in the adult rat dorsal horn following section of a neighbouring peripheral nerve. *J Comp Neurol.* 1997;380(1):95-104.

126. Moore KA, Kohno T, Karchewski LA, Scholz J, Baba H, Woolf CJ. Partial peripheral nerve injury promotes a selective loss of GABAergic inhibition in the superficial dorsal horn of the spinal cord. *J Neurosci.* 2002;22(15):6724-6731.

127. Boadas-Vaello P, Castany S, Homs J, Alvarez-Perez B, Deulofeu M, Verdu E. Neuroplasticity of ascending and descending pathways after somatosensory system injury: reviewing knowledge to identify neuropathic pain therapeutic targets. *Spinal Cord.* 2016;54(5):330-340.

128. Ellis A, Bennett DL. Neuroinflammation and the generation of neuropathic pain. *Br J Anaesth.* 2013;111(1):26-37.

129. Bouhassira D, Attal N. Diagnosis and assessment of neuropathic pain: the saga of clinical tools. *Pain.* 2011;152(3 Suppl):S74-83.

130. Chang VT, Janjan N, Jain S, Chau C. Update in cancer pain syndromes. *J Palliat Med.* 2006;9(6):1414-1434.

131. Bouhassira D, Attal N, Fermanian J, et al. Development and validation of the Neuropathic Pain Symptom Inventory. *Pain.* 2004;108(3):248-257.

132. Attal N, Fermanian C, Fermanian J, Lanteri-Minet M, Alchaar H, Bouhassira D. Neuropathic pain: are there distinct subtypes depending on the aetiology or anatomical lesion? *Pain.* 2008;138(2):343-353.

133. Attal N, Bouhassira D, Baron R, et al. Assessing symptom profiles in neuropathic pain clinical trials: can it improve outcome? *Eur J Pain.* 2011;15(5):441-443.

134. Elliot K, Foley KM. Neurologic pain syndromes in patients with cancer. In: Portenoy RK, ed. *Pain: Mechanisms and Syndromes, Neurologic Clinics.* Vol 7. Philadelphia, PA: Saunders; 1989:333-360.

135. Fallon MT. Neuropathic pain in cancer. *Br J Anaesth.* 2013;111(1):105-111.

136. Urch CE, Dickenson AH. Neuropathic pain in cancer. *Eur J Cancer*. 2008;44(8):1091-1096.

137. Hausheer FH, Schilsky RL, Bain S, Berghorn EJ, Lieberman F. Diagnosis, management, and evaluation of chemotherapy-induced peripheral neuropathy. *Semin Oncol*. 2006;33(1):15-49.

138. Gilron I, Bailey JM, Tu D, Holden RR, Jackson AC, Houlden RL. Nortriptyline and gabapentin, alone and in combination for neuropathic pain: a double-blind, randomised controlled crossover trial. *Lancet*. 2009;374(9697):1252-1261.

139. Jones RC, 3rd, Lawson E, Backonja M. Managing neuropathic pain. *Med Clin North Am*. 2016;100(1):151-167.

140. Beal BR, Wallace MS. An overview of pharmacologic management of chronic pain. *Med Clin North Am*. 2016;100(1):65-79.

141. Pereira J. Management of bone pain. In: Portenoy RK, Bruera E, eds. *Topics in Palliative Care*. Vol 3. New York, NY: Oxford University Press; 1998:79-116.

142. Frisaldi E, Piedimonte A, Benedetti F. Placebo and nocebo effects: a complex interplay between psychological factors and neurochemical networks. *Am J Clin Hypn*. 2015;57(3):267-284.

143. Carlino E, Pollo A, Benedetti F. The placebo in practice: how to use it in clinical routine. *Curr Opin Support Palliat Care*. 2012;6(2):220-225.

144. Benedetti F. Placebo analgesia. *Neurol Sci*. 2006;27 Suppl 2:S100-102.

145. Colloca L. Placebo, nocebo, and learning mechanisms. *Handb Exp Pharmacol*. 2014;225:17-35.

146. Colloca L, Grillon C. Understanding placebo and nocebo responses for pain management. *Curr Pain Headache Rep*. 2014;18(6):419.

147. Colloca L, Miller FG. The nocebo effect and its relevance for clinical practice. *Psychosom Med*. 2011;73(7):598-603.

148. Colloca L, Benedetti F. Placebos and painkillers: is mind as real as matter? *Nat Rev Neurosci*. 2005;6(7):545-552.

149. Benedetti F, Mayberg HS, Wager TD, Stohler CS, Zubieta JK. Neurobiological mechanisms of the placebo effect. *J Neurosci*. 2005;25(45):10390-10402.

150. Hoffman GA, Harrington A, Fields HL. Pain and the placebo: what we have learned. *Perspect Biol Med*. 2005;48(2):248-265.

151. Eippert F, Bingel U, Schoell ED, et al. Activation of the opioidergic descending pain control system underlies placebo analgesia. *Neuron*. 2009;63(4):533-543.

152. Benedetti F. The opposite effects of the opiate antagonist naloxone and the cholecystokinin antagonist proglumide on placebo analgesia. *Pain*. 1996;64(3):535-543.

153. Posner J, Burke CA. The effects of naloxone on opiate and placebo analgesia in healthy volunteers. *Psychopharmacology (Berl)*. 1985;87(4):468-472.

154. Goldstein A, Grevert P. Placebo analgesia, endorphins, and naloxone. *Lancet*. 1978;2(8104-5):1385.

155. Levine JD, Gordon NC, Fields HL. The mechanism of placebo analgesia. *Lancet*. 1978;2(8091):654-657.

156. Walwyn WM, Chen W, Kim H, et al. Sustained suppression of hyperalgesia during latent sensitization by mu-, delta-, and kappa-opioid receptors and alpha2A adrenergic receptors: role of constitutive activity. *J Neurosci*. 2016;36(1):204-221.

157. Pereira MP, Donahue RR, Dahl JB, Werner M, Taylor BK, Werner MU. Endogenous opioid-masked latent pain sensitization: studies from mouse to human. *PLoS One*. 2015;10(8):e0134441.

158. Pacheco-Lopez G, Engler H, Niemi MB, Schedlowski M. Expectations and associations that heal: immunomodulatory placebo effects and its neurobiology. *Brain Behav Immun*. 2006;20(5):430-446.

159. Wager TD, Rilling JK, Smith EE, et al. Placebo-induced changes in FMRI in the anticipation and experience of pain. *Science*. 2004;303(5661):1162-1167.

160. Benedetti A, Pollo A, Maggi G, et al. Placebo analgesia: from physiological mechanisms to clinical implications. *Proceedings of the 10th Wold Confress on Pain 2003*. 2003;24:315-323.

161. Benedetti F, Rainero I, Pollo A. New insights into placebo analgesia. *Curr Opin Anaesthesiol.* 2003;16(5):515-519.

162. Levine JD, Gordon NC. Influence of the method of drug administration on analgesic response. *Nature.* 1984;312(5996):755-756.

163. Colloca L, Benedetti F. Nocebo hyperalgesia: how anxiety is turned into pain. *Curr Opin Anaesthesiol.* 2007;20(5):435-439.

164. Flaten MA, Simonsen T, Olsen H. Drug-related information generates placebo and nocebo responses that modify the drug response. *Psychosom Med.* 1999;61(2):250-255.

165. Barsky AJ, Saintfort R, Rogers MP, Borus JF. Nonspecific medication side effects and the nocebo phenomenon. *JAMA.* 2002;287(5):622-627.

166. Oftedal G, Straume A, Johnsson A, Stovner LJ. Mobile phone headache: a double blind, sham-controlled provocation study. *Cephalalgia.* 2007;27(5):447-455.

167. Benedetti F, Amanzio M. The neurobiology of placebo analgesia: from endogenous opioids to cholecystokinin. *Prog Neurobiol.* 1997;52(2):109-125.

168. Benedetti F, Amanzio M, Vighetti S, Asteggiano G. The biochemical and neuroendocrine bases of the hyperalgesic nocebo effect. *J Neurosci.* 2006;26(46):12014-12022.

169. Dy SM, Asch SM, Naeim A, Sanati H, Walling A, Lorenz KA. Evidence-based standards for cancer pain management. *J Clin Oncol.* 2008;26(23):3879-3885.

170. Portenoy RK. Treatment of cancer pain. *Lancet.* 2011;377(9784):2236-2247.

171. Weinstein SM. Nonmalignant pain. In: Walsh DA, Caraceni AT, Fainsinger R, eds. *Palliative Medicine.* 1st ed. Philadelphia, PA: Saunders Elsevier; 2008:931-934.

172. Hicks CL, von Baeyer CL, Spafford PA, van Korlaar I, Goodenough B. The Faces Pain Scale-Revised: toward a common metric in pediatric pain measurement. *Pain.* 2001;93(2):173-183.

173. Hockenberry MJ. *Wong's Essentials of Pediatric Nursing.* 7th ed. St. Louis, MO: Mosby; 2005.

174. Jones KR, Vojir CP, Hutt E, Fink R. Determining mild, moderate, and severe pain equivalency across pain-intensity tools in nursing home residents. *J Rehabil Res Dev.* 2007;44(2):305-314.

175. Holen JC, Hjermstad MJ, Loge JH, et al. Pain assessment tools: is the content appropriate for use in palliative care? *J Pain Symptom Manage.* 2006;32(6):567-580.

176. Melzack R. The McGill Pain Questionnaire: major properties and scoring methods. *Pain.* 1975;1(3):277-299.

177. Bruera E, Kuehn N, Miller MJ, Selmser P, Macmillan K. The Edmonton Symptom Assessment System (ESAS): a simple method for the assessment of palliative care patients. *J Palliat Care.* 1991;7(2):6-9.

178. Wilkie DJ, Ezenwa MO, Yao Y, et al. Pain intensity and misconceptions among hospice patients with cancer and their caregivers: status after 2 decades. *Am J Hosp Palliat Care.* 2017;34(4):318-324.

179. Jacobsen R, Moldrup C, Christrup L, Sjogren P. Patient-related barriers to cancer pain management: a systematic exploratory review. *Scand J Caring Sci.* 2009;23(1):190-208.

180. Passik SD. Issues in long-term opioid therapy: unmet needs, risks, and solutions. *Mayo Clin Proc.* 2009;84(7):593-601.

181. Passik S, Kirsh KL. Chemical coping: the clinical middle ground. In: Smith HS, Passik S, eds. *Pain and Chemical Dependency.* New York: Oxford University Press; 2008.

182. Lawlor P, Walker P, Bruera E, Mitchell S. Severe opioid toxicity and somatization of psychosocial distress in a cancer patient with a background of chemical dependence. *J Pain Symptom Manage.* 1997;13(6):356-361.

183. Passik SD, Kirsh KL, Donaghy KB, Portenoy RK. Pain and aberrant drug-related behaviors in medically ill patients with and without histories of substance abuse. *Clin J Pain.* 2006;22(2):173-181.

184. Del Fabbro E. Assessment and management of chemical coping in patients with cancer. *J Clin Oncol.* 2014;32(16):1734-1738.

185. Kwon JH, Tanco K, Hui D, Reddy A, Bruera E. Chemical coping versus pseudoaddiction in patients with cancer pain. *Palliat Support Care.* 2014;12(5):413-417.

186. Kwon JH, Tanco K, Park JC, et al. Frequency, predictors, and medical record documentation of chemical coping among advanced cancer patients. *Oncologist.* 2015;20(6):692-697.

187. Brown RL, Rounds LA. Conjoint screening questionnaires for alcohol and other drug abuse: criterion validity in a primary care practice. *Wis Med J.* 1995;94(3):135-140.

188. Koyyalagunta D, Bruera E, Aigner C, Nusrat H, Driver L, Novy D. Risk stratification of opioid misuse among patients with cancer pain using the SOAPP-SF. *Pain Med.* 2013;14(5):667-675.

189. Webster LR, Webster RM. Predicting aberrant behaviors in opioid-treated patients: preliminary validation of the Opioid Risk Tool. *Pain Med.* 2005;6(6):432-442.

190. Weinstein SM. Physical examination of the patient in pain. In: Ashburn M, ed. *Management of Pain.* New York: Churchill Livingston; 1998:17-25.

191. Desbiens NA, Mueller-Rizner N. How well do surrogates assess the pain of seriously ill patients? *Crit Care Med.* 2000;28(5):1347-1352.

192. Allen RS, Haley WE, Small BJ, McMillan SC. Pain reports by older hospice cancer patients and family caregivers: the role of cognitive functioning. *Gerontologist.* 2002;42(4):507-514.

193. Redinbaugh EM, Baum A, DeMoss C, Fello M, Arnold R. Factors associated with the accuracy of family caregiver estimates of patient pain. *J Pain Symptom Manage.* 2002;23(1):31-38.

194. Gelinas C, Fillion L, Puntillo KA, Viens C, Fortier M. Validation of the critical-care pain observation tool in adult patients. *Am J Crit Care.* 2006;15(4):420-427.

195. Voepel-Lewis T, Zanotti J, Dammeyer JA, Merkel S. Reliability and validity of the face, legs, activity, cry, consolability behavioral tool in assessing acute pain in critically ill patients. *Am J Crit Care.* 2010;19(1):55-61; quiz 62.

196. Puntillo K, Pasero C, Li D, et al. Evaluation of pain in ICU patients. *Chest.* 2009;135(4):1069-1074.

197. Reddy SK, Weinstein SM. Medical decision-making in a patient with a history of cancer and chronic non-malignant pain. *Clin J Pain.* 1995;11(3):242-246.

198. Piovesan EJ. Diagnostic headache criteria and instruments. In: Herndon RM, ed. *Handbook of Neurologic Rating Scales.* 2nd ed. New York: Demos; 2006:297-345.

199. Morley-Forster P. Prevalence of neuropathic pain and need for treatment. *Pain Research & Management.* 2006;11(Suppl. A):5A-10A.

200. Dworkin RH, Backonja M, Rowbotham MC, et al. Advances in neuropathic pain: diagnosis, mechanisms, and treatment recommendations. *Arch Neurol.* 2003;60(11):1524-1534.

201. Ferris FD, Bruera E, Cherny N, et al. Palliative cancer care a decade later: accomplishments, the need, next steps—from the American Society of Clinical Oncology. *J Clin Oncol.* 2009;27(18):3052-3058.

202. Falkmer U, Jarhult J, Wersall P, Cavallin-Stahl E. A systematic overview of radiation therapy effects in skeletal metastases. *Acta Oncol.* 2003;42(5-6):620-633.

203. Tanvetyanon T, Soares HP, Djulbegovic B, Jacobsen PB, Bepler G. A systematic review of quality of life associated with standard chemotherapy regimens for advanced non-small cell lung cancer. *J Thorac Oncol.* 2007;2(12):1091-1097.

204. Cherny NI, Baselga J, de Conno F, Radbruch L. Formulary availability and regulatory barriers to accessibility of opioids for cancer pain in Europe: a report from the ESMO/EAPC Opioid Policy Initiative. *Ann Oncol.* 2010;21(3):615-626.

205. Swarm R, Abernethy AP, Anghelescu DL, et al. Adult cancer pain. *J Natl Compr Canc Netw.* 2010;8(9):1046-1086.

206. Swarm RA. The management of pain in patients with cancer. *J Natl Compr Canc Netw.* 2013;11(5 Suppl):702-704.

207. World Health Organization. *Cancer Pain Relief with a Guide to Opioid Availability.* 2nd ed. Geneva, Switzerland: World Health Organization; 1996.

208. Bandieri E, Romero M, Ripamonti CI, et al. Randomized trial of low-dose morphine versus weak opioids in moderate cancer pain. *J Clin Oncol.* 2016;34(5):436-442.

209. Vargas-Schaffer G. Is the WHO analgesic ladder still valid? Twenty-four years of experience. *Can Fam Physician.* 2010;56(6):514-517, e202-515.

210. Bhatnagar S, Gupta M. Evidence-based clinical practice guidelines for interventional pain management in cancer pain. *Indian J Palliat Care.* 2015;21(2):137-147.

211. Pasternak GW. Opiate pharmacology and relief of pain. *J Clin Oncol.* 2014;32(16):1655-1661.

212. Butour JL, Moisand C, Mazarguil H, Mollereau C, Meunier JC. Recognition and activation of the opioid receptor-like ORL 1 receptor by nociceptin, nociceptin analogs and opioids. *Eur J Pharmacol.* 1997;321(1):97-103.

213. Fioravanti B, Vanderah TW. The ORL-1 receptor system: are there opportunities for antagonists in pain therapy? *Curr Top Med Chem.* 2008;8(16):1442-1451.

214. Kirkpatrick DR, McEntire DM, Hambsch ZJ, et al. Therapeutic basis of clinical pain modulation. *Clin Transl Sci.* 2015;8(6):848-856.

215. Fletcher D, Martinez V. Opioid-induced hyperalgesia in patients after surgery: a systematic review and a meta-analysis. *Br J Anaesth.* 2014;112(6):991-1004.

216. Chen L, Malarick C, Seefeld L, Wang S, Houghton M, Mao J. Altered quantitative sensory testing outcome in subjects with opioid therapy. *Pain.* 2009;143(1-2):65-70.

217. Zhang Y, Ahmed S, Vo T, et al. Increased pain sensitivity in chronic pain subjects on opioid therapy: a cross-sectional study using quantitative sensory testing. *Pain Med.* 2015;16(5):911-922.

218. Wang H, Akbar M, Weinsheimer N, Gantz S, Schiltenwolf M. Longitudinal observation of changes in pain sensitivity during opioid tapering in patients with chronic low-back pain. *Pain Med.* 2011;12(12):1720-1726.

219. Carullo V, Fitz-James I, Delphin E. Opioid-induced hyperalgesia: a diagnostic dilemma. *J Pain Palliat Care Pharmacother.* 2015;29(4):378-384.

220. Mao J. Clinical diagnosis of opioid-induced hyperalgesia. *Reg Anesth Pain Med.* 2015;40(6):663-664.

221. Yi P, Pryzbylkowski P. Opioid induced hyperalgesia. *Pain Med.* 2015;16 Suppl 1:S32-36.

222. Chu LF, Dairmont J, Zamora AK, Young CA, Angst MS. The endogenous opioid system is not involved in modulation of opioid-induced hyperalgesia. *J Pain.* 2011;12(1):108-115.

223. Kapitzke D, Vetter I, Cabot PJ. Endogenous opioid analgesia in peripheral tissues and the clinical implications for pain control. *Ther Clin Risk Manag.* 2005;1(4):279-297.

224. Lee M, Silverman SM, Hansen H, Patel VB, Manchikanti L. A comprehensive review of opioid-induced hyperalgesia. *Pain Physician.* 2011;14(2):145-161.

225. Grace PM, Ramos KM, Rodgers KM, et al. Activation of adult rat CNS endothelial cells by opioid-induced toll-like receptor 4 (TLR4) signaling induces proinflammatory, biochemical, morphological, and behavioral sequelae. *Neuroscience.* 2014;280:299-317.

226. Hutchinson MR, Zhang Y, Shridhar M, et al. Evidence that opioids may have toll-like receptor 4 and MD-2 effects. *Brain Behav Immun.* 2010;24(1):83-95.

227. Hutchinson MR, Coats BD, Lewis SS, et al. Proinflammatory cytokines oppose opioid-induced acute and chronic analgesia. *Brain Behav Immun.* 2008;22(8):1178-1189.

228. Lee C, Lee HW, Kim JN. Effect of oral pregabalin on opioid-induced hyperalgesia in patients undergoing laparo-endoscopic single-site urologic surgery. *Korean J Anesthesiol.* 2013;64(1):19-24.

229. Stoicea N, Russell D, Weidner G, et al. Opioid-induced hyperalgesia in chronic pain patients and the mitigating effects of gabapentin. *Front Pharmacol.* 2015;6:104.

230. Wei X, Wei W. Role of gabapentin in preventing fentanyl- and morphine-withdrawal-induced hyperalgesia in rats. *J Anesth.* 2012;26(2):236-241.

231. Compton P, Kehoe P, Sinha K, Torrington MA, Ling W. Gabapentin improves cold-pressor pain responses in methadone-maintained patients. *Drug Alcohol Depend.* 2010;109(1-3):213-219.

232. Van Elstraete AC, Sitbon P, Mazoit JX, Benhamou D. Gabapentin prevents delayed and long-lasting hyperalgesia induced by fentanyl in rats. *Anesthesiology.* 2008;108(3):484-494.

233. Dunbar SA, Karamian I, Zhang J. Ketorolac prevents recurrent withdrawal induced hyperalgesia but does not inhibit tolerance to spinal morphine in the rat. *Eur J Pain.* 2007;11(1):1-6.

234. Cormie PJ, Nairn M, Welsh J. Control of pain in adults with cancer: summary of SIGN guidelines. *BMJ.* 2008;337:a2154.

235. Trescot AM. Review of the role of opioids in cancer pain. *J Natl Compr Canc Netw.* 2010;8(9):1087-1094.

236. Green E, Zwaal C, Beals C, et al. Cancer-related pain management: a report of evidence-based recommendations to guide practice. *Clin J Pain.* 2010;26(6):449-462.

237. Dworkin RH, O'Connor AB, Backonja M, et al. Pharmacologic management of neuropathic pain: evidence-based recommendations. *Pain.* 2007;132(3):237-251.

238. Caraceni A, Hanks G, Kaasa S, et al. Use of opioid analgesics in the treatment of cancer pain: evidence-based recommendations from the EAPC. *Lancet Oncol.* 2012;13(2):e58-68.

239. Kurita GP, Kaasa S, Sjogren P. Spinal opioids in adult patients with cancer pain: a systematic review: a European Palliative Care Research Collaborative (EPCRC) opioid guidelines project. *Palliat Med.* 2011;25(5):560-577.

240. Mercadante S, Caraceni A. Conversion ratios for opioid switching in the treatment of cancer pain: a systematic review. *Palliat Med.* 2011;25(5):504-515.

241. Klepstad P, Kaasa S, Borchgrevink PC. Starting step III opioids for moderate to severe pain in cancer patients: dose titration: a systematic review. *Palliat Med.* 2011;25(5):424-430.

242. Caraceni A, Pigni A, Brunelli C. Is oral morphine still the first choice opioid for moderate to severe cancer pain? A systematic review within the European Palliative Care Research Collaborative guidelines project. *Palliat Med.* 2011;25(5):402-409.

243. Schmidt-Hansen M, Bromham N, Taubert M, Arnold S, Hilgart JS. Buprenorphine for treating cancer pain. *Cochrane Database Syst Rev.* 2015;3:CD009596.

244. Cuomo A, Russo G, Esposito G, Forte CA, Connola M, Marcassa C. Efficacy and gastrointestinal tolerability of oral oxycodone/naloxone combination for chronic pain in outpatients with cancer: an observational study. *Am J Hosp Palliat Care.* 2014;31(8):867-876.

245. Blagden M, Hafer J, Duerr H, Hopp M, Bosse B. Long-term evaluation of combined prolonged-release oxycodone and naloxone in patients with moderate-to-severe chronic pain: pooled analysis of extension phases of two Phase III trials. *Neurogastroenterol Motil.* 2014;26(12):1792-1801.

246. Mercadante S, Ferrera P, Adile C. High doses of oxycodone-naloxone combination may provide poor analgesia. *Support Care Cancer.* 2011;19(9):1471-1472.

247. Setnik B, Sommerville K, Pixton G, Webster L. Extended-release morphine sulfate and naltrexone hydrochloride: naltrexone associated effects in chronic pain patients and recreational opioid users. *J Pain.* 2014;15:S6.

248. Raffa RB, Taylor R, Jr., Pergolizzi JV, Jr. Sequestered naltrexone in sustained release morphine or oxycodone—a way to inhibit illicit use? *Expert Opin Drug Saf.* 2014;13(2):181-190.

249. Cordery SF, Taverner A, Ridzwan IE, et al. A non-rewarding, non-aversive buprenorphine/naltrexone combination attenuates drug-primed reinstatement to cocaine and morphine in rats in a conditioned place preference paradigm. *Addict Biol.* 2014;19(4):575-586.

250. Schneider JP, Matthews M, Jamison RN. Abuse-deterrent and tamper-resistant opioid formulations: what is their role in addressing prescription opioid abuse? *CNS Drugs.* 2010;24(10):805-810.

251. Walter C, Knothe C, Lotsch J. Abuse-deterrent opioid formulations: pharmacokinetic and pharmacodynamic considerations. *Clin Pharmacokinet.* 2016;55(7):751-767.

252. Hwang CS, Chang HY, Alexander GC. Impact of abuse-deterrent OxyContin on prescription opioid utilization. *Pharmacoepidemiol Drug Saf.* 2015;24(2):197-204.

253. Lotsch J, Rohrbacher M, Schmidt H, Doehring A, Brockmoller J, Geisslinger G. Can extremely low or high morphine formation from codeine be predicted prior to therapy initiation? *Pain.* 2009;144(1-2):119-124.

254. Klepstad P, Dale O, Kaasa S, et al. Influences on serum concentrations of morphine, M6G and M3G during routine clinical drug monitoring: a prospective survey in 300 adult cancer patients. *Acta Anaesthesiol Scand.* 2003;47(6):725-731.

255. Davis M. Cholestasis and endogenous opioids: liver disease and exogenous opioid pharmacokinetics. *Clin Pharmacokinet.* 2007;46(10):825-850.

256. Bosilkovska M, Walder B, Besson M, Daali Y, Desmeules J. Analgesics in patients with hepatic impairment: pharmacology and clinical implications. *Drugs.* 2012;72(12):1645-1669.

257. O'Connor NR, Corcoran AM. End-stage renal disease: symptom management and advance care planning. *Am Fam Physician.* 2012;85(7):705-710.

258. Suno M, Endo Y, Nishie H, Kajizono M, Sendo T, Matsuoka J. Refractory cachexia is associated with increased plasma concentrations of fentanyl in cancer patients. *Ther Clin Risk Manag.* 2015;11:751-757.

259. Heiskanen T, Matzke S, Haakana S, Gergov M, Vuori E, Kalso E. Transdermal fentanyl in cachectic cancer patients. *Pain.* 2009;144(1-2):218-222.

260. Naito T, Tashiro M, Ishida T, Ohnishi K, Kawakami J. Cancer cachexia raises the plasma concentration of oxymorphone through the reduction of CYP3A but not CYP2D6 in oxycodone-treated patients. *J Clin Pharmacol.* 2013;53(8):812-818.

261. Naito T, Tashiro M, Yamamoto K, Ohnishi K, Kagawa Y, Kawakami J. Impact of cachexia on pharmacokinetic disposition of and clinical responses to oxycodone in cancer patients. *Eur J Clin Pharmacol.* 2012;68(10):1411-1418.

262. Knotkova H, Fine PG, Portenoy RK. Opioid rotation: the science and the limitations of the equianalgesic dose table. *J Pain Symptom Manage.* 2009;38(3):426-439.

263. Fine PG, Portenoy RK, Ad Hoc Expert Panel on Evidence Review and Guidelines for Opioid Rotation. Establishing "best practices" for opioid rotation: conclusions of an expert panel. *J Pain Symptom Manage.* 2009;38(3):418-425.

264. Maltoni M, Scarpi E, Modonesi C, et al. A validation study of the WHO analgesic ladder: a two-step vs three-step strategy. *Support Care Cancer.* 2005;13(11):888-894.

265. Gammaitoni AR, Fine P, Alvarez N, McPherson ML, Bergmark S. Clinical application of opioid equianalgesic data. *Clin J Pain.* 2003;19(5):286-297.

266. Breitbart W, Chandler S, Eagel B, et al. An alternative algorithm for dosing transdermal fentanyl for cancer-related pain. *Oncology (Williston Park)*. 2000;14(5):695-705; discussion 705, 709-617.

267. Modesto-Lowe V, Brooks D, Petry N. Methadone deaths: risk factors in pain and addicted populations. *J Gen Intern Med*.25(4):305-309.

268. Bruera E, Sweeney C. Methadone use in cancer patients with pain: a review. *J Palliat Med*. 2002;5(1):127-138.

269. Iribarne C, Dreano Y, Bardou LG, Menez JF, Berthou F. Interaction of methadone with substrates of human hepatic cytochrome P450 3A4. *Toxicology*. 1997;117(1):13-23.

270. Reddy S, Hui D, El Osta B, et al. The effect of oral methadone on the QTc interval in advanced cancer patients: a prospective pilot study. *J Palliat Med*. 2010;13(1):33-38.

271. Demarie D, Marletta G, Imazio M, et al. Cardiovascular-associated disease in an addicted population: an observation study. *J Cardiovasc Med*. 2011;12(1):51-54.

272. Keller GA, Ponte ML, Di Girolamo G. Other drugs acting on nervous system associated with QT-interval prolongation. *Current drug safety*. 2010;5(1):105-111.

273. King S, Forbes K, Hanks GW, Ferro CJ, Chambers EJ. A systematic review of the use of opioid medication for those with moderate to severe cancer pain and renal impairment: a European Palliative Care Research Collaborative opioid guidelines project. *Palliat Med*. 2011;25(5):525-552.

274. Bryson J, Tamber A, Seccareccia D, Zimmermann C. Methadone for treatment of cancer pain. *Curr Oncol Rep*. 2006;8(4):282-288.

275. Sandoval JA, Furlan AD, Mailis-Gagnon A. Oral methadone for chronic noncancer pain: a systematic literature review of reasons for administration, prescription patterns, effectiveness, and side effects. *Clin J Pain*. 2005;21(6):503-512.

276. Bruera E, Palmer JL, Bosnjak S, et al. Methadone versus morphine as a first-line strong opioid for cancer pain: a randomized, double-blind study. *J Clin Oncol*. 2004;22(1):185-192.

277. Mercadante S, Porzio G, Ferrera P, et al. Sustained-release oral morphine versus transdermal fentanyl and oral methadone in cancer pain management. *Eur J Pain*. 2008;12(8):1040-1046.

278. Mathew P, Storey P. Subcutaneous methadone in terminally ill patients: manageable local toxicity. *J Pain Symptom Manage*. 1999;18(1):49-52.

279. Chou R, Cruciani RA, Fiellin DA, et al. Methadone safety: a clinical practice guideline from the American Pain Society and College on Problems of Drug Dependence, in collaboration with the Heart Rhythm Society. *J Pain*. 2014;15(4):321-337.

280. Chou R, Weimer MB, Dana T. Methadone overdose and cardiac arrhythmia potential: findings from a review of the evidence for an American Pain Society and College on Problems of Drug Dependence clinical practice guideline. *J Pain*. 2014;15(4):338-365.

281. Zeppetella G. Impact and management of breakthrough pain in cancer. *Curr Opin Support Palliat Care*. 2009;3(1):1-6.

282. Aronoff GM, Brennan MJ, Pritchard DD, Ginsberg B. Evidence-based oral transmucosal fentanyl citrate (OTFC) dosing guidelines. *Pain Med*. 2005;6(4):305-314.

283. Coluzzi PH, Schwartzberg L, Conroy JD, et al. Breakthrough cancer pain: a randomized trial comparing oral transmucosal fentanyl citrate (OTFC) and morphine sulfate immediate release (MSIR). *Pain*. 2001;91(1-2):123-130.

284. Mercadante S. Pharmacotherapy for breakthrough cancer pain. *Drugs*. 2012;72(2):181-190.

285. Mercadante S, Ferrera P, Adile C, Casuccio A. Fentanyl buccal tablets for breakthrough pain in highly tolerant cancer patients: preliminary data on the proportionality between breakthrough pain dose and background dose. *J Pain Symptom Manage*. 2011;42(3):464-469.

286. Douglas C, Clarke M, Alexander S, Khatun M. A tertiary hospital audit of opioids and sedatives administered in the last 24 h of life. *Intern Med J.* 2016;46(3):325-331.

287. Kestenbaum MG, Vilches AO, Messersmith S, et al. Alternative routes to oral opioid administration in palliative care: a review and clinical summary. *Pain Med.* 2014;15(7):1129-1153.

288. Davis MP, Walsh D, LeGrand SB, Naughton M. Symptom control in cancer patients: the clinical pharmacology and therapeutic role of suppositories and rectal suspensions. *Support Care Cancer.* 2002;10(2):117-138.

289. Tassinari D, Sartori S, Tamburini E, et al. Transdermal fentanyl as a front-line approach to moderate-severe pain: a meta-analysis of randomized clinical trials. *J Palliat Care.* 2009;25(3):172-180.

290. Gulaboski R, Cordeiro MN, Milhazes N, et al. Evaluation of the lipophilic properties of opioids, amphetamine-like drugs, and metabolites through electrochemical studies at the interface between two immiscible solutions. *Anal Biochem.* 2007;361(2):236-243.

291. Staats PS, Markowitz J, Schein J. Incidence of constipation associated with long-acting opioid therapy: a comparative study. *South Med J.* 2004;97(2):129-134.

292. Aluminium-containing transdermal patches: a risk of burns. *Prescrire Int.* 2007;16(92):246.

293. Gordon DB, Stevenson KK, Griffie J, Muchka S, Rapp C, Ford-Roberts K. Opioid equianalgesic calculations. *J Palliat Med.* 1999;2(2):209-218.

294. Skaer TL. Transdermal opioids for cancer pain. *Health Qual Life Outcomes.* 2006;4:24.

295. Davis MP. Twelve reasons for considering buprenorphine as a frontline analgesic in the management of pain. *J Support Oncol.* 2012;10(6):209-219.

296. Hand CW, Sear JW, Uppington J, Ball MJ, McQuay HJ, Moore RA. Buprenorphine disposition in patients with renal impairment: single and continuous dosing, with special reference to metabolites. *Br J Anaesth.* 1990;64(3):276-282.

297. Hanks GW, Conno F, Cherny N, et al. Morphine and alternative opioids in cancer pain: the EAPC recommendations. *Br J Cancer.* 2001;84(5):587-593.

298. Campiglia L, Cappellini I, Consales G, et al. Premedication with sublingual morphine sulphate in abdominal surgery. *Clin Drug Investig.* 2009;29 Suppl 1:25-30.

299. Kokki H, Rasanen I, Lasalmi M, et al. Comparison of oxycodone pharmacokinetics after buccal and sublingual administration in children. *Clin Pharmacokinet.* 2006;45(7):745-754.

300. Wilkinson TJ, Robinson BA, Begg EJ, Duffull SB, Ravenscroft PJ, Schneider JJ. Pharmacokinetics and efficacy of rectal versus oral sustained-release morphine in cancer patients. *Cancer Chemother Pharmacol.* 1992;31(3):251-254.

301. Bruera E, MacEachern T, Ripamonti C, Hanson J. Subcutaneous morphine for dyspnea in cancer patients. *Ann Intern Med.* 1993;119(9):906-907.

302. Dale O, Sheffels P, Kharasch ED. Bioavailabilities of rectal and oral methadone in healthy subjects. *Br J Clin Pharmacol.* 2004;58(2):156-162.

303. Storey P, Trumble M. Rectal doxepin and carbamazepine therapy in patients with cancer. *N Engl J Med.* 1992;327(18):1318-1319.

304. Pikwer A, Akeson J, Lindgren S. Complications associated with peripheral or central routes for central venous cannulation. *Anaesthesia.* 2012;67(1):65-71.

305. Wilcock A, Jacob JK, Charlesworth S, Harris E, Gibbs M, Allsop H. Drugs given by a syringe driver: a prospective multicentre survey of palliative care services in the UK. *Palliat Med.* 2006;20(7):661-664.

306. Grass JA. Patient-controlled analgesia. *Anesth Analg.* 2005;101(5 Suppl):S44-61.

307. Johnson FK, Ciric S, Boudriau S, Kisicki JC, Stauffer J. The relative bioavailability of morphine sulfate and naltrexone hydrochloride extended release capsules (EMBEDA®) and an extended release morphine sulfate capsule formulation (KADIAN®) in healthy adults under fasting conditions. *Am J Ther*. 2011;18(1):2-8.

308. Sloan PA. Neuraxial pain relief for intractable cancer pain. *Curr Pain Headache Rep*. 2007;11(4):283-289.

309. Smith TJ, Staats PS, Deer T, et al. Randomized clinical trial of an implantable drug delivery system compared with comprehensive medical management for refractory cancer pain: impact on pain, drug-related toxicity, and survival. *J Clin Oncol*. 2002;20(19):4040-4049.

310. Cohen SP, Dragovich A. Intrathecal analgesia. *Med Clin North Am*. 2007;91(2):251-270.

311. Burton AW, Rajagopal A, Shah HN, et al. Epidural and intrathecal analgesia is effective in treating refractory cancer pain. *Pain Med*. 2004;5(3):239-247.

312. Prager J, Deer T, Levy R, et al. Best practices for intrathecal drug delivery for pain. *Neuromodulation*. 2014;17(4):354-372; discussion 372.

313. Horlocker TT, Burton AW, Connis RT, et al. Practice guidelines for the prevention, detection, and management of respiratory depression associated with neuraxial opioid administration. *Anesthesiology*. 2009;110(2):218-230.

314. Enzmann DR, Pelc NJ. Normal flow patterns of intracranial and spinal cerebrospinal fluid defined with phase-contrast cine MR imaging. *Radiology*. 1991;178(2):467-474.

315. Greitz D. Cerebrospinal fluid circulation and associated intracranial dynamics. A radiologic investigation using MR imaging and radionuclide cisternography. *Acta Radiol Suppl*. 1993;386:1-23.

316. Bernards CM. Cerebrospinal fluid and spinal cord distribution of baclofen and bupivacaine during slow intrathecal infusion in pigs. *Anesthesiology*. 2006;105(1):169-178.

317. van der Plas AA, Marinus J, Eldabe S, Buchser E, van Hilten JJ. The lack of efficacy of different infusion rates of intrathecal baclofen in complex regional pain syndrome: a randomized, double-blind, crossover study. *Pain Med*. 2011;12(3):459-465.

318. Perruchoud C, Eldabe S, Durrer A, et al. Effects of flow rate modifications on reported analgesia and quality of life in chronic pain patients treated with continuous intrathecal drug therapy. *Pain Med*. 2011;12(4):571-576.

319. Bernards CM. Recent insights into the pharmacokinetics of spinal opioids and the relevance to opioid selection. *Curr Opin Anaesthesiol*. 2004;17(5):441-447.

320. Deer TR, Prager J, Levy R, et al. Polyanalgesic Consensus Conference—2012: recommendations on trialing for intrathecal (intraspinal) drug delivery: report of an interdisciplinary expert panel. *Neuromodulation*. 2012;15(5):420-435; discussion 435.

321. Ummenhofer WC, Arends RH, Shen DD, Bernards CM. Comparative spinal distribution and clearance kinetics of intrathecally administered morphine, fentanyl, alfentanil, and sufentanil. *Anesthesiology*. 2000;92(3):739-753.

322. Bernards CM. Understanding the physiology and pharmacology of epidural and intrathecal opioids. *Best Pract Res Clin Anaesthesiol*. 2002;16(4):489-505.

323. Schug SA, Saunders D, Kurowski I, Paech MJ. Neuraxial drug administration: a review of treatment options for anaesthesia and analgesia. *CNS Drugs*. 2006;20(11):917-933.

324. Stewart J, Kellett N, Castro D. The central nervous system and cardiovascular effects of levobupivacaine and ropivacaine in healthy volunteers. *Anesth Analg*. 2003;97(2):412-416, table of contents.

325. Eisenach JC, DeKock M, Klimscha W. alpha(2)-adrenergic agonists for regional anesthesia—a clinical review of clonidine (1984-1995). *Anesthesiology*. 1996;85(3):655-674.

326. Mercadante S, Calderone L, Sapio M, Serretta R, Passafiume M. Comfort sedation by clonidine during intrathecal anaesthesia for cesarean section. *Br J Anaesth*. 1996;76:A337-A337.

327.  Belhadj Amor M, Draief A, Ouezini R, et al. 30 microg intrathecal clonidine prolongs labour analgesia, but increases the incidence of hypotension and abnormal foetal heart rate patterns. *Ann Fr Anesth Reanim.* 2007;26(11):916-920.

328.  Deer TR, Smith HS, Burton AW, et al. Comprehensive consensus based guidelines on intrathecal drug delivery systems in the treatment of pain caused by cancer pain. *Pain Physician.* 2011;14(3):E283-312.

329.  Pope JE, Deer TR. Ziconotide: a clinical update and pharmacologic review. *Expert Opin Pharmacother.* 2013;14(7):957-966.

330.  Fainsinger RL, Nekolaichuk CL, Lawlor PG, Neumann CM, Hanson J, Vigano A. A multicenter study of the revised Edmonton Staging System for classifying cancer pain in advanced cancer patients. *J Pain Symptom Manage.* 2005;29(3):224-237.

331.  Mercadante S, Bruera E. Opioid switching: a systematic and critical review. *Cancer Treat Rev.* 2006;32(4):304-315.

332.  Baldini A, Von Korff M, Lin EH. A review of potential adverse effects of long-term opioid therapy: a practitioner's guide. *Prim Care Companion CNS Disord.* 2012;14(3).

333.  Solomon DH, Rassen JA, Glynn RJ, et al. The comparative safety of opioids for nonmalignant pain in older adults. *Arch Intern Med.* 2010;170(22):1979-1986.

334.  Solomon DH, Rassen JA, Glynn RJ, Lee J, Levin R, Schneeweiss S. The comparative safety of analgesics in older adults with arthritis. *Arch Intern Med.* 2010;170(22):1968-1976.

335.  Carman WJ, Su S, Cook SF, Wurzelmann JI, McAfee A. Coronary heart disease outcomes among chronic opioid and cyclooxygenase-2 users compared with a general population cohort. *Pharmacoepidemiol Drug Saf.* 2011;20(7):754-762.

336.  Vuong C, Van Uum SH, O'Dell LE, Lutfy K, Friedman TC. The effects of opioids and opioid analogs on animal and human endocrine systems. *Endocr Rev.* 2010;31(1):98-132.

337.  Katz N, Mazer NA. The impact of opioids on the endocrine system. *Clin J Pain.* 2009;25(2):170-175.

338.  Huang G, Travison T, Maggio M, Edwards RR, Basaria S. Effects of testosterone replacement on metabolic and inflammatory markers in men with opioid-induced androgen deficiency. *Clin Endocrinol (Oxf).* 2016;85(2):232-238.

339.  Fanoe S, Jensen GB, Sjogren P, Korsgaard MP, Grunnet M. Oxycodone is associated with dose-dependent QTc prolongation in patients and low-affinity inhibiting of hERG activity in vitro. *Br J Clin Pharmacol.* 2009;67(2):172-179.

340.  Raffa RB, Burmeister JJ, Yuvasheva E, Pergolizzi JV, Jr. QTc interval prolongation by d-propoxyphene: what about other analgesics? *Expert Opin Pharmacother.* 2012;13(10):1397-1409.

341.  Katchman AN, McGroary KA, Kilborn MJ, et al. Influence of opioid agonists on cardiac human ether-a-go-go-related gene K(+) currents. *J Pharmacol Exp Ther.* 2002;303(2):688-694.

342.  Baker JR, Best AM, Pade PA, McCance-Katz EF. Effect of buprenorphine and antiretroviral agents on the QT interval in opioid-dependent patients. *Ann Pharmacother.* 2006;40(3):392-396.

343.  Fanoe S, Hvidt C, Ege P, Jensen GB. Syncope and QT prolongation among patients treated with methadone for heroin dependence in the city of Copenhagen. *Heart.* 2007;93(9):1051-1055.

344.  Anchersen K, Clausen T, Gossop M, Hansteen V, Waal H. Prevalence and clinical relevance of corrected QT interval prolongation during methadone and buprenorphine treatment: a mortality assessment study. *Addiction.* 2009;104(6):993-999.

345.  Athanasos P, Farquharson AL, Compton P, Psaltis P, Hay J. Electrocardiogram characteristics of methadone and buprenorphine maintained subjects. *J Addict Dis.* 2008;27(3):31-35.

346.  Sittl R. Transdermal buprenorphine in cancer pain and palliative care. *Palliat Med.* 2006;20 Suppl 1:s25-30.

347. Griessinger N, Sittl R, Likar R. Transdermal buprenorphine in clinical practice—a post-marketing surveillance study in 13,179 patients. *Curr Med Res Opin.* 2005;21(8):1147-1156.

348. Sittl R, Griessinger N, Likar R. Analgesic efficacy and tolerability of transdermal buprenorphine in patients with inadequately controlled chronic pain related to cancer and other disorders: a multicenter, randomized, double-blind, placebo-controlled trial. *Clin Ther.* 2003;25(1):150-168.

349. Sorge J, Sittl R. Transdermal buprenorphine in the treatment of chronic pain: results of a phase III, multicenter, randomized, double-blind, placebo-controlled study. *Clin Ther.* 2004;26(11):1808-1820.

350. Lindgren L, Saarnivaara L, Klemola UM. Protection by fentanyl against cardiac dysrhythmias during induction of anaesthesia. *Eur J Anaesthesiol.* 1987;4(4):229-233.

351. Chang DJ, Kweon TD, Nam SB, et al. Effects of fentanyl pretreatment on the QTc interval during propofol induction. *Anaesthesia.* 2008;63(10):1056-1060.

352. Shah RR. Drug-induced prolongation of the QT interval: why the regulatory concern? *Fundam Clin Pharmacol.* 2002;16(2):119-124.

353. Skjervold B, Bathen J, Spigset O. Methadone and the QT interval: relations to the serum concentrations of methadone and its enantiomers (R)-methadone and (S)-methadone. *J Clin Psychopharmacol.* 2006;26(6):687-689.

354. Ehret GB, Voide C, Gex-Fabry M, et al. Drug-induced long QT syndrome in injection drug users receiving methadone: high frequency in hospitalized patients and risk factors. *Arch Intern Med.* 2006;166(12):1280-1287.

355. Sagie A, Larson MG, Goldberg RJ, Bengtson JR, Levy D. An improved method for adjusting the QT interval for heart rate (the Framingham Heart Study). *Am J Cardiol.* 1992;70(7):797-801.

356. Pearson EC, Woosley RL. QT prolongation and torsades de pointes among methadone users: reports to the FDA spontaneous reporting system. *Pharmacoepidemiol Drug Saf.* 2005;14(11):747-753.

357. Glare P, Walsh D, Sheehan D. The adverse effects of morphine: a prospective survey of common symptoms during repeated dosing for chronic cancer pain. *Am J Hosp Palliat Care.* 2006;23(3):229-235.

358. McNicol E. Opioid side effects and their treatment in patients with chronic cancer and noncancer pain. *J Pain Palliat Care Pharmacother.* 2008;22(4):270-281.

359. Mercadante S, Calderone L, Villari P, et al. The use of pilocarpine in opioid-induced xerostomia. *Palliat Med.* 2000;14(6):529-531.

360. White ID, Hoskin PJ, Hanks GW, Bliss JM. Morphine and dryness of the mouth. *BMJ.* 1989;298(6682):1222-1223.

361. Tammela T, Kontturi M, Lukkarinen O. Postoperative urinary retention. I. Incidence and predisposing factors. *Scand J Urol Nephrol.* 1986;20(3):197-201.

362. O'Riordan JA, Hopkins PM, Ravenscroft A, Stevens JD. Patient-controlled analgesia and urinary retention following lower limb joint replacement: prospective audit and logistic regression analysis. *Eur J Anaesthesiol.* 2000;17(7):431-435.

363. Rawal N, Mollefors K, Axelsson K, Lingardh G, Widman B. An experimental study of urodynamic effects of epidural morphine and of naloxone reversal. *Anesth Analg.* 1983;62(7):641-647.

364. Malinovsky JM, Le Normand L, Lepage JY, et al. The urodynamic effects of intravenous opioids and ketoprofen in humans. *Anesth Analg.* 1998;87(2):456-461.

365. Rosow CE, Gomery P, Chen TY, Stefanovich P, Stambler N, Israel R. Reversal of opioid-induced bladder dysfunction by intravenous naloxone and methylnaltrexone. *Clin Pharmacol Ther.* 2007;82(1):48-53.

366. Holzer P, Ahmedzai SH, Niederle N, et al. Opioid-induced bowel dysfunction in cancer-related pain: causes, consequences, and a novel approach for its management. *J Opioid Manag.* 2009;5(3):145-151.

367. Mancini I, Bruera E. Constipation in advanced cancer patients. *Support Care Cancer.* 1998;6(4):356-364.

368. Nelson AD, Camilleri M. Opioid-induced constipation: advances and clinical guidance. *Ther Adv Chronic Dis.* 2016;7(2):121-134.

369. Gaertner J, Siemens W, Camilleri M, et al. Definitions and outcome measures of clinical trials regarding opioid-induced constipation: a systematic review. *J Clin Gastroenterol.* 2015;49(1):9-16.

370. Shook JE, Lemcke PK, Gehrig CA, Hruby VJ, Burks TF. Antidiarrheal properties of supraspinal mu and delta and peripheral mu, delta and kappa opioid receptors: inhibition of diarrhea without constipation. *J Pharmacol Exp Ther.* 1989;249(1):83-90.

371. Choi YS, Billings JA. Opioid antagonists: a review of their role in palliative care, focusing on use in opioid-related constipation. *J Pain Symptom Manage.* 2002;24(1):71-90.

372. Tuteja AK, Biskupiak J, Stoddard GJ, Lipman AG. Opioid-induced bowel disorders and narcotic bowel syndrome in patients with chronic non-cancer pain. *Neurogastroenterol Motil.* 2010;22(4):424-430, e496.

373. Becker G, Galandi D, Blum HE. Peripherally acting opioid antagonists in the treatment of opiate-related constipation: a systematic review. *J Pain Symptom Manage.* 2007;34(5):547-565.

374. Mehta N, O'Connell K, Giambrone GP, Baqai A, Diwan S. Efficacy of methylnaltrexone for the treatment of opiod-induced constipation: a meta-analysis and systematic review. *Postgrad Med.* 2016;128(3):282-289.

375. Slatkin NE, Lynn R, Su C, Wang W, Israel RJ. Characterization of abdominal pain during methylnaltrexone treatment of opioid-induced constipation in advanced illness: a post hoc analysis of two clinical trials. *J Pain Symptom Manage.* 2011;42(5):754-760.

376. Jansen JP, Lorch D, Langan J, et al. A randomized, placebo-controlled phase 3 trial (Study SB-767905/012) of alvimopan for opioid-induced bowel dysfunction in patients with non-cancer pain. *J Pain.* 2011;12(2):185-193.

377. Cryer B, Mareya S, Joswick T, et al. Spontaneous bowel movement frequency is improved over 12 weeks of lubiprostone therapy in opioid-induced constipation patients regardless of gender, age, or race: pooled analysis of three well-controlled studies. *Am J Gastroenterol.* 2013;108:S567.

378. Spierings EL, Brewer RP, Rauck RL, Losch-Beridon T, Mareya SM. Lubiprostone for opioid-induced constipation does not interfere with opioid analgesia in patients with chronic noncancer pain. *Pain Pract.* 2017;17(3):312-319.

379. Lubiprostone (Amitiza) for opioid-induced constipation. *Med Lett Drugs Ther.* 2013;55(1418):47-48.

380. Chey WD, Webster L, Sostek M, Lappalainen J, Barker PN, Tack J. Naloxegol for opioid-induced constipation in patients with noncancer pain. *N Engl J Med.* 2014;370(25):2387-2396.

381. Ford AC, Brenner DM, Schoenfeld PS. Efficacy of pharmacological therapies for the treatment of opioid-induced constipation: systematic review and meta-analysis. *Am J Gastroenterol.* 2013;108(10):1566-1574; quiz 1575.

382. Stern EJ. Chronic, progressive, bibasilar infiltrates in a woman with constipation. *Chest.* 1992;102(1):263-265.

383. Paraskevaides EC. Fatal lipid pneumonia and liquid paraffin. *Br J Clin Pract.* 1990;44(11):509-510.

384. Becker GL. The case against mineral oil. *Am J Dig Dis.* 1952;19(11):344-348.

385. Sussman G, Shurman J, Creed MR, et al. Intravenous ondansetron for the control of opioid-induced nausea and vomiting. International S3AA3013 Study Group. *Clin Ther.* 1999;21(7):1216-1227.

386. Hornby PJ. Central neurocircuitry associated with emesis. *Am J Med.* 2001;111 Suppl 8A:106S-112S.

387. Barnes NM, Bunce KT, Naylor RJ, Rudd JA. The actions of fentanyl to inhibit drug-induced emesis. *Neuropharmacology.* 1991;30(10):1073-1083.

388. Scotto di Fazano C, Vergne P, Grilo RM, Bertin P, Bonnet C, Treves R. [Preventive therapy for nausea and vomiting in patients on opioid therapy for non-malignant pain in rheumatology]. *Therapie.* 2002;57(5):446-449.

389. Holden JE, Jeong Y, Forrest JM. The endogenous opioid system and clinical pain management. *AACN Clin Issues.* 2005;16(3):291-301.

390. Freye E, Latasch L. Development of opioid tolerance—molecular mechanisms and clinical consequences. *Anasthesiol Intensivmed Notfallmed Schmerzther.* 2003;38(1):14-26.

391. Portenoy RK, Farrar JT, Backonja MM, et al. Long-term use of controlled-release oxycodone for noncancer pain: results of a 3-year registry study. *Clin J Pain.* 2007;23(4):287-299.

392. Campora E, Merlini L, Pace M, et al. The incidence of narcotic-induced emesis. *J Pain Symptom Manage.* 1991;6(7):428-430.

393. Hardy J, Daly S, McQuade B, et al. A double-blind, randomised, parallel group, multinational, multicentre study comparing a single dose of ondansetron 24 mg p.o. with placebo and metoclopramide 10 mg t.d.s. p.o. in the treatment of opioid-induced nausea and emesis in cancer patients. *Support Care Cancer.* 2002;10(3):231-236.

394. Harnett MJ, O'Rourke N, Walsh M, Carabuena JM, Segal S. Transdermal scopolamine for prevention of intrathecal morphine-induced nausea and vomiting after cesarean delivery. *Anesth Analg.* 2007;105(3):764-769.

395. Okamoto Y, Tsuneto S, Matsuda Y, et al. A retrospective chart review of the antiemetic effectiveness of risperidone in refractory opioid-induced nausea and vomiting in advanced cancer patients. *J Pain Symptom Manage.* 2007;34(2):217-222.

396. Maxwell LG, Kaufmann SC, Bitzer S, et al. The effects of a small-dose naloxone infusion on opioid-induced side effects and analgesia in children and adolescents treated with intravenous patient-controlled analgesia: a double-blind, prospective, randomized, controlled study. *Anesth Analg.* 2005;100(4):953-958.

397. Harris JD. Management of expected and unexpected opioid-related side effects. *Clin J Pain.* 2008;24 Suppl 10:S8-s13.

398. McNicol E, Horowicz-Mehler N, Fisk RA, et al. Management of opioid side effects in cancer-related and chronic noncancer pain: a systematic review. *J Pain.* 2003;4(5):231-256.

399. Vestergaard P, Rejnmark L, Mosekilde L. Anxiolytics, sedatives, antidepressants, neuroleptics and the risk of fracture. *Osteoporos Int.* 2006;17(6):807-816.

400. Miller M, Sturmer T, Azrael D, Levin R, Solomon DH. Opioid analgesics and the risk of fractures in older adults with arthritis. *J Am Geriatr Soc.* 2011;59(3):430-438.

401. Takkouche B, Montes-Martinez A, Gill SS, Etminan M. Psychotropic medications and the risk of fracture: a meta-analysis. *Drug Saf.* 2007;30(2):171-184.

402. Shorr RI, Griffin MR, Daugherty JR, Ray WA. Opioid analgesics and the risk of hip fracture in the elderly: codeine and propoxyphene. *J Gerontol.* 1992;47(4):M111-115.

403. Saunders KW, Dunn KM, Merrill JO, et al. Relationship of opioid use and dosage levels to fractures in older chronic pain patients. *J Gen Intern Med.* 2010;25(4):310-315.

404. Vestergaard P, Rejnmark L, Mosekilde L. Fracture risk associated with the use of morphine and opiates. *J Intern Med.* 2006;260(1):76-87.

405. Kamal-Bahl SJ, Stuart BC, Beers MH. Propoxyphene use and risk for hip fractures in older adults. *Am J Geriatr Pharmacother.* 2006;4(3):219-226.

406. Gotthardt F, Huber C, Thierfelder C, et al. Bone mineral density and its determinants in men with opioid dependence. *J Bone Miner Metab.* 2016.

407. Coluzzi F, Pergolizzi J, Raffa RB, Mattia C. The unsolved case of "bone-impairing analgesics": the endocrine effects of opioids on bone metabolism. *Ther Clin Risk Manag.* 2015;11:515-523.

408. Merza Z. Chronic use of opioids and the endocrine system. *Horm Metab Res.* 2010;42(9):621-626.

409. Daniell HW. DHEAS deficiency during consumption of sustained-action prescribed opioids: evidence for opioid-induced inhibition of adrenal androgen production. *J Pain.* 2006;7(12):901-907.

410. Facchinetti F, Comitini G, Petraglia F, Volpe A, Genazzani AR. Reduced estriol and dehydroepiandrosterone sulphate plasma levels in methadone-addicted pregnant women. *Eur J Obstet Gynecol Reprod Biol.* 1986;23(1-2):67-73.

411. Gudin JA, Laitman A, Nalamachu S. Opioid related endocrinopathy. *Pain Med.* 2015;16 Suppl 1:S9-15.

412. Benyamin R, Trescot AM, Datta S, et al. Opioid complications and side effects. *Pain Physician.* 2008;11(2 Suppl):S105-120.

413. Roberts LJ, Finch PM, Pullan PT, Bhagat CI, Price LM. Sex hormone suppression by intrathecal opioids: a prospective study. *Clin J Pain.* 2002;18(3):144-148.

414. Woody G, Luborsky L, McLellan A, O'Brien C. Psychotherapy for substance abuse. *NIDA Res Monogr.* 1988;90:162-167.

415. Rubinstein AL, Carpenter DM, Minkoff JR. Hypogonadism in men with chronic pain linked to the use of long-acting rather than short-acting opioids. *Clin J Pain.* 2013;29(10):840-845.

416. Daniell HW. Hypogonadism in men consuming sustained-action oral opioids. *J Pain.* 2002;3(5):377-384.

417. Daniell HW. Narcotic-induced hypogonadism during therapy for heroin addiction. *J Addict Dis.* 2002;21(4):47-53.

418. Daniell HW. Hypothyroidism: a frequent event after radiotherapy for patients with head and neck carcinoma. *Cancer.* 2002;95(3):673-674; author reply 674.

419. Bliesener N, Albrecht S, Schwager A, Weckbecker K, Lichtermann D, Klingmuller D. Plasma testosterone and sexual function in men receiving buprenorphine maintenance for opioid dependence. *J Clin Endocrinol Metab.* 2005;90(1):203-206.

420. Hallinan R, Byrne A, Agho K, McMahon C, Tynan P, Attia J. Erectile dysfunction in men receiving methadone and buprenorphine maintenance treatment. *J Sex Med.* 2008;5(3):684-692.

421. Hallinan R, Byrne A, Agho K, McMahon CG, Tynan P, Attia J. Hypogonadism in men receiving methadone and buprenorphine maintenance treatment. *Int J Androl.* 2009;32(2):131-139.

422. Basaria S. Testosterone levels for evaluation of androgen deficiency. *JAMA.* 2015;313(17):1749-1750.

423. Basaria S, Travison TG, Alford D, et al. Effects of testosterone replacement in men with opioid-induced androgen deficiency: a randomized controlled trial. *Pain.* 2015;156(2):280-288.

424. Long JB, Holaday JW. Blood-brain barrier: endogenous modulation by adrenal-cortical function. *Science.* 1985;227(4694):1580-1583.

425. Miner MM, Khera M, Bhattacharya RK, Blick G, Kushner H. Baseline data from the TRiUS registry: symptoms and comorbidities of testosterone deficiency. *Postgrad Med.* 2011;123(3):17-27.

426. Ananthakrishnan P, Cohen DB, Xu DZ, Lu Q, Feketeova E, Deitch EA. Sex hormones modulate distant organ injury in both a trauma/hemorrhagic shock model and a burn model. *Surgery.* 2005;137(1):56-65.

427. Ensrud KE, Blackwell T, Mangione CM, et al. Central nervous system active medications and risk for fractures in older women. *Arch Intern Med.* 2003;163(8):949-957.

428. Daniell HW. Opioid contribution to decreased cortisol levels in critical care patients. *Arch Surg.* 2008;143(12):1147-1148.

429. Daniell HW. Opioid endocrinopathy in women consuming prescribed sustained-action opioids for control of nonmalignant pain. *J Pain.* 2008;9(1):28-36.

430. Abs R, Verhelst J, Maeyaert J, et al. Endocrine consequences of long-term intrathecal administration of opioids. *J Clin Endocrinol Metab.* 2000;85(6):2215-2222.

431. Gold PW, Extein I, Pickar D, Rebar R, Ross R, Goodwin FK. Supression of plasma cortisol in depressed patients by acute intravenous methadone infusion. *Am J Psychiatry.* 1980;137(7):862-863.

432. Bawor M, Dennis BB, Samaan MC, et al. Methadone induces testosterone suppression in patients with opioid addiction. *Sci Rep.* 2014;4:6189.

433. Bhasin S, Cunningham GR, Hayes FJ, et al. Testosterone therapy in men with androgen deficiency syndromes: an Endocrine Society clinical practice guideline. *J Clin Endocrinol Metab.* 2010;95(6):2536-2559.

434. Eichenbaum G, Gohler K, Etropolski M, et al. Does tapentadol affect sex hormone concentrations differently from morphine and oxycodone? An initial assessment and possible implications for opioid-induced androgen deficiency. *J Opioid Manag.* 2015;11(3):211-227.

435. Dandona P, Rosenberg MT. A practical guide to male hypogonadism in the primary care setting. *Int J Clin Pract.* 2010;64(6):682-696.

436. Elliott JA, Horton E, Fibuch EE. The endocrine effects of long-term oral opioid therapy: a case report and review of the literature. *J Opioid Manag.* 2011;7(2):145-154.

437. Sacerdote P. Opioid-induced immunosuppression. *Curr Opin Support Palliat Care.* 2008;2(1):14-18.

438. Sacerdote P. Opioids and the immune system. *Palliat Med.* 2006;20 Suppl 1:s9-15.

439. Sacerdote P, Franchi S, Panerai AE. Non-analgesic effects of opioids: mechanisms and potential clinical relevance of opioid-induced immunodepression. *Curr Pharm Des.* 2012;18(37):6034-6042.

440. Peterson PK, Molitor TW, Chao CC. The opioid-cytokine connection. *J Neuroimmunol.* 1998;83(1-2):63-69.

441. Stephanou A, Fitzharris P, Knight RA, Lightman SL. Characteristics and kinetics of proopiomelanocortin mRNA expression by human leucocytes. *Brain Behav Immun.* 1991;5(4):319-327.

442. Byas-Smith MG, Chapman SL, Reed B, Cotsonis G. The effect of opioids on driving and psychomotor performance in patients with chronic pain. *Clin J Pain.* 2005;21(4):345-352.

443. Emery MJ, Groves CC, Kruse TN, Shi C, Terman GW. Ventilation and the response to hypercapnia after morphine in opioid-naive and opioid-tolerant rats. *Anesthesiology.* 2016;124(4):945-957.

444. Ahmedzai S. New approaches to pain control in patients with cancer. *Eur J Cancer.* 1997;33 Suppl 6:S8-14.

445. Bruera E, Miller MJ, Macmillan K, Kuehn N. Neuropsychological effects of methylphenidate in patients receiving a continuous infusion of narcotics for cancer pain. *Pain.* 1992;48(2):163-166.

446. Wilwerding MB, Loprinzi CL, Mailliard JA, et al. A randomized, crossover evaluation of methylphenidate in cancer patients receiving strong narcotics. *Support Care Cancer.* 1995;3(2):135-138.

447. Reissig JE, Rybarczyk AM. Pharmacologic treatment of opioid-induced sedation in chronic pain. *Ann Pharmacother.* 2005;39(4):727-731.

448. Schatzberg AF. Opioids in psychiatric disorders: back to the future? *Am J Psychiatry.* 2015:appiajp201515101354.

449. Yovell Y, Bar G, Mashiah M, et al. Ultra-low-dose buprenorphine as a time-limited treatment for severe suicidal ideation: a randomized controlled trial. *Am J Psychiatry.* 2016;173(5):491-498.

450. Mercadante S. Pathophysiology and treatment of opioid-related myoclonus in cancer patients. *Pain.* 1998;74(1):5-9.

451. Lyss AP, Portenoy RK. Strategies for limiting the side effects of cancer pain therapy. *Semin Oncol.* 1997;24(5 Suppl 16):S16-28-34.

452. Dale O, Moksnes K, Kaasa S. European Palliative Care Research Collaborative pain guidelines: opioid switching to improve analgesia or reduce side effects. A systematic review. *Palliat Med.* 2011;25(5):494-503.

453. Cherny N, Ripamonti C, Pereira J, et al. Strategies to manage the adverse effects of oral morphine: an evidence-based report. *J Clin Oncol.* 2001;19(9):2542-2554.

454. Stone P, Minton O. European Palliative Care Research collaborative pain guidelines. Central side-effects management: what is the evidence to support best practice in the management of sedation, cognitive impairment and myoclonus? *Palliat Med.* 2011;25(5):431-441.

455. Eisele JH, Jr., Grigsby EJ, Dea G. Clonazepam treatment of myoclonic contractions associated with high-dose opioids: case report. *Pain.* 1992;49(2):231-232.

456. Vella-Brincat J, Macleod AD. Adverse effects of opioids on the central nervous systems of palliative care patients. *J Pain Palliat Care Pharmacother*. 2007;21(1):15-25.

457. Holtkamp M, Halle A, Meierkord H, Masuhr F. Gabapentin-induced severe myoclonus in a patient with impaired renal function. *J Neurol*. 2006;253(3):382-383.

458. Mercadante S, Villari P, Fulfaro F. Gabapentin for opiod-related myoclonus in cancer patients. *Support Care Cancer*. 2001;9(3):205-206.

459. Asconape J, Diedrich A, DellaBadia J. Myoclonus associated with the use of gabapentin. *Epilepsia*. 2000;41(4):479-481.

460. Hustveit O. Interaction between opioid and muscarinic receptors in the guinea-pig ileum preparation: a mathematical model. *Pharmacol Toxicol*. 1996;78(3):167-173.

461. Gaudreau JD, Gagnon P, Roy MA, Harel F, Tremblay A. Opioid medications and longitudinal risk of delirium in hospitalized cancer patients. *Cancer*. 2007;109(11):2365-2373.

462. Tanaka R, Ishikawa H, Sato T, et al. Incidence of delirium among patients having cancer injected with different opioids for the first time. *Am J Hosp Palliat Care*. 2016;34(6):572-576.

463. Rughooputh N, Griffiths R. Tramadol and delirium. *Anaesthesia*. 2015;70(5):632-633.

464. Slatkin N, Rhiner M. Treatment of opioid-induced delirium with acetylcholinesterase inhibitors: a case report. *J Pain Symptom Manage*. 2004;27(3):268-273.

465. Yue HJ, Guilleminault C. Opioid medication and sleep-disordered breathing. *Med Clin North Am*. 2010;94(3):435-446.

466. Webster LR, Choi Y, Desai H, Webster L, Grant BJ. Sleep-disordered breathing and chronic opioid therapy. *Pain Med*. 2008;9(4):425-432.

467. Mogri M, Desai H, Webster L, Grant BJ, Mador MJ. Hypoxemia in patients on chronic opiate therapy with and without sleep apnea. *Sleep Breath*. 2009;13(1):49-57.

468. Walker JM, Farney RJ, Rhondeau SM, et al. Chronic opioid use is a risk factor for the development of central sleep apnea and ataxic breathing. *J Clin Sleep Med*. 2007;3(5):455-461.

469. Teichtahl H, Wang D, Cunnington D, et al. Ventilatory responses to hypoxia and hypercapnia in stable methadone maintenance treatment patients. *Chest*. 2005;128(3):1339-1347.

470. Feldman JL, Del Negro CA. Looking for inspiration: new perspectives on respiratory rhythm. *Nat Rev Neurosci*. 2006;7(3):232-242.

471. Farney RJ, McDonald AM, Boyle KM, et al. Sleep disordered breathing in patients receiving therapy with buprenorphine/naloxone. *Eur Respir J*. 2013;42(2):394-403.

472. Zaremba S, Shin CH, Hutter MM, et al. Continuous positive airway pressure mitigates opioid-induced worsening of sleep-disordered breathing early after bariatric surgery. *Anesthesiology*. 2016;125(1):92-104.

473. Dunn KM, Saunders KW, Rutter CM, et al. Opioid prescriptions for chronic pain and overdose: a cohort study. *Ann Intern Med*. 2010;152(2):85-92.

474. Boyer EW. Management of opioid analgesic overdose. *N Engl J Med*. 2012;367(2):146-155.

475. Fala L, Welz JA. New perspectives in the treatment of opioid-induced respiratory depression. *Am Health Drug Benefits*. 2015;8(6 Suppl 3):S51-63.

476. Robinson A, Wermeling DP. Intranasal naloxone administration for treatment of opioid overdose. *Am J Health Syst Pharm*. 2014;71(24):2129-2135.

477. van der Schier R, Roozekrans M, van Velzen M, Dahan A, Niesters M. Opioid-induced respiratory depression: reversal by non-opioid drugs. *F1000Prime Rep*. 2014;6:79.

478. Paulozzi LJ, Kilbourne EM, Shah NG, et al. A history of being prescribed controlled substances and risk of drug overdose death. *Pain Med*. 2012;13(1):87-95.

479. Katz NP, Adams EH, Benneyan JC, et al. Foundations of opioid risk management. *Clin J Pain.* 2007;23(2):103-118.

480. Portenoy RK. Acute and chronic pain. In: Ruiz P, Strain, E., ed. *Lowinson & Ruiz's Substance Abuse: A Comprehensive Textbook.* 5th ed. Philadelphia, PA: Lippincott Williams & Wilkins; 2011.

481. Savage SR, Joranson DE, Covington EC, Schnoll SH, Heit HA, Gilson AM. Definitions related to the medical use of opioids: evolution towards universal agreement. *J Pain Symptom Manage.* 2003;26(1):655-667.

482. Portenoy RK. Pain specialists and addiction medicine specialists unite to address critical issues. http://www.ampainsoc.org/library/bulletin/mar99/president.htm. Accessed January 31, 2012.

483. Webster LR, Fine PG. Approaches to improve pain relief while minimizing opioid abuse liability. *J Pain.* 2010;11(7):602-611.

484. Sehgal N, Manchikanti L, Smith HS. Prescription opioid abuse in chronic pain: a review of opioid abuse predictors and strategies to curb opioid abuse. *Pain Physician.* 2012;15(3 Suppl):ES67-92.

485. Robb V. Working on the edge: palliative care for substance users with AIDS. *J Palliat Care.* 1995;11(2):50-53.

486. Kirsh KL, Passik SD. Palliative care of the terminally ill drug addict. *Cancer Invest.* 2006;24(4):425-431.

487. Payne R, Anderson E, Arnold R, et al. A rose by any other name: pain contracts/agreements. *Am J Bioeth.* 2010;10(11):5-12.

488. Morita T, Tsunoda J, Inoue S, Chihara S. Effects of high dose opioids and sedatives on survival in terminally ill cancer patients. *J Pain Symptom Manage.* 2001;21(4):282-289.

489. Portenoy RK, Sibirceva U, Smout R, et al. Opioid use and survival at the end of life: a survey of a hospice population. *J Pain Symptom Manage.* 2006;32(6):532-540.

490. Davis MP. Recent development in therapeutics for breakthrough pain. *Expert Rev Neurother.* 2010;10(5):757-773.

491. Davis MP, Weissman DE, Arnold RM. Opioid dose titration for severe cancer pain: a systematic evidence-based review. *J Palliat Med.* 2004;7(3):462-468.

492. Axelsson B, Borup S. Is there an additive analgesic effect of paracetamol at step 3? A double-blind randomized controlled study. *Palliat Med.* 2003;17(8):724-725.

493. Stockler M, Vardy J, Pillai A, Warr D. Acetaminophen (paracetamol) improves pain and well-being in people with advanced cancer already receiving a strong opioid regimen: a randomized, double-blind, placebo-controlled cross-over trial. *J Clin Oncol.* 2004;22(16):3389-3394.

494. Israel FJ, Parker G, Charles M, Reymond L. Lack of benefit from paracetamol (acetaminophen) for palliative cancer patients requiring high-dose strong opioids: a randomized, double-blind, placebo-controlled, crossover trial. *J Pain Symptom Manage.* 2010;39(3):548-554.

495. Cubero DI, del Giglio A. Early switching from morphine to methadone is not improved by acetaminophen in the analgesia of oncologic patients: a prospective, randomized, double-blind, placebo-controlled study. *Support Care Cancer.* 2010;18(2):235-242.

496. US Food and Drug Administration. FDA Drug Safety Communication: Prescription Acetaminophen Products to be Limited to 325 mg Per Dosage Unit; Boxed Warning Will Highlight Potential for Severe Liver Failure. http://www.fda.gov/Drugs/DrugSafety/ucm239821.htm. Accessed July 15, 2017.

497. Chen Y, Dong H, Thompson DC, Shertzer HG, Nebert DW, Vasiliou V. Glutathione defense mechanism in liver injury: insights from animal models. *Food Chem Toxicol.* 2013;60:38-44.

498. Waring WS. Novel acetylcysteine regimens for treatment of paracetamol overdose. *Ther Adv Drug Saf.* 2012;3(6):305-315.

499. Manchanda A, Cameron C, Robinson G. Beware of paracetamol use in alcohol abusers: a potential cause of acute liver injury. *N Z Med J.* 2013;126(1383):80-84.

500. Holt EW, DeMartini S, Davern TJ. Acute liver failure due to acetaminophen poisoning in patients with prior weight loss surgery: a case series. *J Clin Gastroenterol.* 2015;49(9):790-793.

501. Jatox A, Carr DB, Payne R, et al. *Management of Cancer Pain. Clinical Practice Guideline 9. ACHPR Publication 94-0592.* Rockville, MD: Agency for Health Care Policy and Research, US Department of Health and Human Services, Public Health Survey; 1994.

502. Eisenberg E, Berkey CS, Carr DB, Mosteller F, Chalmers TC. Efficacy and safety of nonsteroidal antiinflammatory drugs for cancer pain: a meta-analysis. *J Clin Oncol.* 1994;12(12):2756-2765.

503. McNicol E, Strassels SA, Goudas L, Lau J, Carr DB. NSAIDS or paracetamol, alone or combined with opioids, for cancer pain. *Cochrane Database Syst Rev.* 2005(1):CD005180.

504. Hinz B, Renner B, Brune K. Drug insight: cyclo-oxygenase-2 inhibitors—a critical appraisal. *Nat Clin Pract Rheumatol.* 2007;3(10):552-560.

505. Lanza FL, Chan FK, Quigley EM. Guidelines for prevention of NSAID-related ulcer complications. *Am J Gastroenterol.* 2009;104(3):728-738.

506. Scheiman JM. Prevention of NSAID-induced ulcers. *Curr Treat Options Gastroenterol.* 2008;11(2):125-134.

507. Lazzaroni M, Porro GB. Management of NSAID-induced gastrointestinal toxicity: focus on proton pump inhibitors. *Drugs.* 2009;69(1):51-69.

508. Farkouh ME, Greenberg BP. An evidence-based review of the cardiovascular risks of nonsteroidal anti-inflammatory drugs. *Am J Cardiol.* 2009;103(9):1227-1237.

509. Lussier D, Portenoy, RK. Adjuvant analgesics in pain management. In: Hanks G, Cherny, N, Christakis, N, Kaasa S, Fallon M, Portenoy RK, eds. *Oxford Textbook of Palliative Medicine.* 4th ed. Oxford: Oxford University Press; 2010:706-733.

510. Mercadante S, Portenoy RK. Opioid poorly-responsive cancer pain. Part 3. Clinical strategies to improve opioid responsiveness. *J Pain Symptom Manage.* 2001;21(4):338-354.

511. Della Cuna GR, Pellegrini A, Piazzi M. Effect of methylprednisolone sodium succinate on quality of life in preterminal cancer patients: a placebo-controlled, multicenter study. The Methylprednisolone Preterminal Cancer Study Group. *Eur J Cancer Clin Oncol.* 1989;25(12):1817-1821.

512. Tannock I, Gospodarowicz M, Meakin W, Panzarella T, Stewart L, Rider W. Treatment of metastatic prostatic cancer with low-dose prednisone: evaluation of pain and quality of life as pragmatic indices of response. *J Clin Oncol.* 1989;7(5):590-597.

513. Mercadante SL, Berchovich M, Casuccio A, Fulfaro F, Mangione S. A prospective randomized study of corticosteroids as adjuvant drugs to opioids in advanced cancer patients. *Am J Hosp Palliat Care.* 2007;24(1):13-19.

514. George R, Jeba J, Ramkumar G, Chacko AG, Leng M, Tharyan P. Interventions for the treatment of metastatic extradural spinal cord compression in adults. *Cochrane Database Syst Rev.* 2008(4):CD006716.

515. Verdu B, Decosterd I, Buclin T, Stiefel F, Berney A. Antidepressants for the treatment of chronic pain. *Drugs.* 2008;68(18):2611-2632.

516. Onghena P, Van Houdenhove B. Antidepressant-induced analgesia in chronic non-malignant pain: a meta-analysis of 39 placebo-controlled studies. *Pain.* 1992;49(2):205-219.

517. Collins SL, Moore RA, McQuayHj, Wiffen P. Antidepressants and anticonvulsants for diabetic neuropathy and postherpetic neuralgia: a quantitative systematic review. *J Pain Symptom Manage.* 2000;20(6):449-458.

518. Saarto T, Wiffen PJ. Antidepressants for neuropathic pain. *Cochrane Database Syst Rev.* 2007(4):CD005454.

519. Sindrup SH, Gram LF, Skjold T, Froland A, Beck-Nielsen H. Concentration-response relationship in imipramine treatment of diabetic neuropathy symptoms. *Clin Pharmacol Ther.* 1990;47(4):509-515.

520. Max MB, Lynch SA, Muir J, Shoaf SE, Smoller B, Dubner R. Effects of desipramine, amitriptyline, and fluoxetine on pain in diabetic neuropathy. *N Engl J Med.* 1992;326(19):1250-1256.

521. Sindrup SH, Bach FW, Madsen C, Gram LF, Jensen TS. Venlafaxine versus imipramine in painful polyneuropathy: a randomized, controlled trial. *Neurology.* 2003;60(8):1284-1289.

522. Rowbotham MC, Goli V, Kunz NR, Lei D. Venlafaxine extended release in the treatment of painful diabetic neuropathy: a double-blind, placebo-controlled study. *Pain.* 2004;110(3):697-706.

523. Arnold LM, Rosen A, Pritchett YL, et al. A randomized, double-blind, placebo-controlled trial of duloxetine in the treatment of women with fibromyalgia with or without major depressive disorder. *Pain.* 2005;119(1-3):5-15.

524. Wernicke JF, Pritchett YL, D'Souza DN, et al. A randomized controlled trial of duloxetine in diabetic peripheral neuropathic pain. *Neurology.* 2006;67(8):1411-1420.

525. Sindrup SH, Gram LF, Brosen K, Eshoj O, Mogensen EF. The selective serotonin reuptake inhibitor paroxetine is effective in the treatment of diabetic neuropathy symptoms. *Pain.* 1990;42(2):135-144.

526. Sindrup SH, Bjerre U, Dejgaard A, Brosen K, Aaes-Jorgensen T, Gram LF. The selective serotonin reuptake inhibitor citalopram relieves the symptoms of diabetic neuropathy. *Clin Pharmacol Ther.* 1992;52(5):547-552.

527. Semenchuk MR, Sherman S, Davis B. Double-blind, randomized trial of bupropion SR for the treatment of neuropathic pain. *Neurology.* 2001;57(9):1583-1588.

528. Derry S, Wiffen PJ, Aldington D, Moore RA. Nortriptyline for neuropathic pain in adults. *Cochrane Database Syst Rev.* 2015;1:Cd011209.

529. Hearn L, Moore RA, Derry S, Wiffen PJ, Phillips T. Desipramine for neuropathic pain in adults. *Cochrane Database Syst Rev.* 2014(9):Cd011003.

530. Eisenach JC, DuPen S, Dubois M, Miguel R, Allin D. Epidural clonidine analgesia for intractable cancer pain. The Epidural Clonidine Study Group. *Pain.* 1995;61(3):391-399.

531. Malanga GA, Gwynn MW, Smith R, Miller D. Tizanidine is effective in the treatment of myofascial pain syndrome. *Pain Physician.* 2002;5(4):422-432.

532. Arain SR, Ruehlow RM, Uhrich TD, Ebert TJ. The efficacy of dexmedetomidine versus morphine for postoperative analgesia after major inpatient surgery. *Anesth Analg.* 2004;98(1):153-158, table of contents.

533. Grotenhermen F. Cannabinoids. *Curr Drug Targets CNS Neurol Disord.* 2005;4(5):507-530.

534. Ben-Shabat S, Fride E, Sheskin T, et al. An entourage effect: inactive endogenous fatty acid glycerol esters enhance 2-arachidonoyl-glycerol cannabinoid activity. *Eur J Pharmacol.* 1998;353(1):23-31.

535. Noyes R, Jr., Brunk SF, Avery DA, Canter AC. The analgesic properties of delta-9-tetrahydrocannabinol and codeine. *Clin Pharmacol Ther.* 1975;18(1):84-89.

536. Noyes R, Jr., Brunk SF, Baram DA, Canter A. Analgesic effect of delta-9-tetrahydrocannabinol. *J Clin Pharmacol.* 1975;15(2-3):139-143.

537. Martin-Sanchez E, Furukawa TA, Taylor J, Martin JL. Systematic review and meta-analysis of cannabis treatment for chronic pain. *Pain Med.* 2009;10(8):1353-1368.

538. Johnson JR, Burnell-Nugent M, Lossignol D, Ganae-Motan ED, Potts R, Fallon MT. Multicenter, double-blind, randomized, placebo-controlled, parallel-group study of the efficacy, safety, and tolerability of THC:CBD extract and THC extract in patients with intractable cancer-related pain. *J Pain Symptom Manage.* 2010;39(2):167-179.

539. Portenoy RK, Ganae-Motan ED, Allende S, et al. Nabiximols for opioid-treated cancer patients with poorly-controlled chronic pain: a randomized, placebo-controlled, graded-dose trial. *J Pain.* 2012;13(5):438-449.

540. Hoggart B, Ratcliffe S, Ehler E, et al. A multicentre, open-label, follow-on study to assess the long-term maintenance of effect, tolerance and safety of THC/CBD oromucosal spray in the management of neuropathic pain. *J Neurol.* 2015;262(1):27-40.

541. Galer BS, Rowbotham MC, Perander J, Friedman E. Topical lidocaine patch relieves postherpetic neuralgia more effectively than a vehicle topical patch: results of an enriched enrollment study. *Pain.* 1999;80(3):533-538.

542. Rowbotham MC, Davies PS, Fields HL. Topical lidocaine gel relieves postherpetic neuralgia. *Ann Neurol.* 1995;37(2):246-253.

543. Stow PJ, Glynn CJ, Minor B. EMLA cream in the treatment of post-herpetic neuralgia. Efficacy and pharmacokinetic profile. *Pain.* 1989;39(3):301-305.

544. Barbano RL, Herrmann DN, Hart-Gouleau S, Pennella-Vaughan J, Lodewick PA, Dworkin RH. Effectiveness, tolerability, and impact on quality of life of the 5% lidocaine patch in diabetic polyneuropathy. *Arch Neurol.* 2004;61(6):914-918.

545. Gammaitoni AR, Galer BS, Onawola R, Jensen MP, Argoff CE. Lidocaine patch 5% and its positive impact on pain qualities in osteoarthritis: results of a pilot 2-week, open-label study using the Neuropathic Pain Scale. *Curr Med Res Opin.* 2004;20 Suppl 2:S13-19.

546. Gammaitoni AR, Alvarez NA, Galer BS. Pharmacokinetics and safety of continuously applied lidocaine patches 5%. *Am J Health Syst Pharm.* 2002;59(22):2215-2220.

547. Knotkova H, Pappagallo M, Szallasi A. Capsaicin (TRPV1 Agonist) therapy for pain relief: farewell or revival? *Clin J Pain.* 2008;24(2):142-154.

548. US Food and Drug Administration. FDA approves new drug treatment for long-term pain relief after shingles attacks. http://www.fda.gov/NewsEvents/Newsroom/PressAnnouncements/2009/ucm191003.htm. Accessed January 31, 2012.

549. Derry S, Conaghan P, Da Silva JA, Wiffen PJ, Moore RA. Topical NSAIDs for chronic musculoskeletal pain in adults. *Cochrane Database Syst Rev.* 2016;4:CD007400.

550. Lin J, Zhang W, Jones A, Doherty M. Efficacy of topical non-steroidal anti-inflammatory drugs in the treatment of osteoarthritis: meta-analysis of randomised controlled trials. *BMJ.* 2004;329(7461):324.

551. Ho KY, Huh BK, White WD, Yeh CC, Miller EJ. Topical amitriptyline versus lidocaine in the treatment of neuropathic pain. *Clin J Pain.* 2008;24(1):51-55.

552. Swarm RA, Anghelescu DL, Bruce JN, et al. NCCN Clinical Practice Guidelines in Oncology (NCCN Guidelines): Adult Cancer Pain. Vol 2.2017. Fort Washington, PA: National Comprehensive Cancer Network; 2017. https://www.nccn.org/professionals/physician_gls/pdf/pain.pdf. Accessed July 15, 2017.

553. Dworkin RH, Kirkpatrick P. Pregabalin. *Nat Rev Drug Discov.* 2005;4(6):455-456.

554. Tzellos TG, Papazisis G, Toulis KA, Sardeli C, Kouvelas D. A2delta ligands gabapentin and pregabalin: future implications in daily clinical practice. *Hippokratia.* 2010;14(2):71-75.

555. Taylor CP, Angelotti T, Fauman E. Pharmacology and mechanism of action of pregabalin: the calcium channel alpha2-delta (alpha2-delta) subunit as a target for antiepileptic drug discovery. *Epilepsy Res.* 2007;73(2):137-150.

556. Moore RA, Wiffen PJ, Derry S, McQuay HJ. Gabapentin for chronic neuropathic pain and fibromyalgia in adults. *Cochrane Database Syst Rev.* 2011(3):CD007938.

557. Alles SR, Smith PA. The anti-allodynic gabapentinoids: myths, paradoxes, and acute effects. *Neuroscientist.* 2016.

558. Wong W, Wallace MS. Determination of the effective dose of pregabalin on human experimental pain using the sequential up-down method. *J Pain.* 2014;15(1):25-31.

559. Guay DR. Pregabalin in neuropathic pain: a more "pharmaceutically elegant" gabapentin? *Am J Geriatr Pharmacother.* 2005;3(4):274-287.

560. Backonja M, Glanzman RL. Gabapentin dosing for neuropathic pain: evidence from randomized, placebo-controlled clinical trials. *Clin Ther.* 2003;25(1):81-104.

561. Papazisis G, Tzachanis D. Pregabalin's abuse potential: a mini review focusing on the pharmacological profile. *Int J Clin Pharmacol Ther.* 2014;52(8):709-716.

562. Schifano F. Misuse and abuse of pregabalin and gabapentin: cause for concern? *CNS Drugs.* 2014;28(6):491-496.

563. Baird CR, Fox P, Colvin LA. Gabapentinoid abuse in order to potentiate the effect of methadone: a survey among substance misusers. *Eur Addict Res.* 2014;20(3):115-118.

564. *Gabapentin for Adults with Neuropathic Pain: A Review of the Clinical Efficacy and Safety.* Ottawa, ON: Canadian Agency for Drugs and Technologies in Health; 2015.

565. Tanenberg RJ, Irving GA, Risser RC, et al. Duloxetine, pregabalin, and duloxetine plus gabapentin for diabetic peripheral neuropathic pain management in patients with inadequate pain response to gabapentin: an open-label, randomized, noninferiority comparison. *Mayo Clin Proc.* 2011;86(7):615-626.

566. Eisenberg E, River Y, Shifrin A, Krivoy N. Antiepileptic drugs in the treatment of neuropathic pain. *Drugs.* 2007;67(9):1265-1289.

567. Wiffen PJ, McQuay HJ, Moore RA. Carbamazepine for acute and chronic pain. *Cochrane Database Syst Rev.* 2005(3):CD005451.

568. Wiffen PJ, Rees J. Lamotrigine for acute and chronic pain. *Cochrane Database Syst Rev.* 2007(2):CD006044.

569. Nasreddine W, Beydoun A. Oxcarbazepine in neuropathic pain. *Expert Opin Investig Drugs.* 2007;16(10):1615-1625.

570. Bendaly EA, Jordan CA, Staehler SS, Rushing DA. Topiramate in the treatment of neuropathic pain in patients with cancer. *Support Cancer Ther.* 2007;4(4):241-246.

571. Wymer JP, Simpson J, Sen D, Bongardt S. Efficacy and safety of lacosamide in diabetic neuropathic pain: an 18-week double-blind placebo-controlled trial of fixed-dose regimens. *Clin J Pain.* 2009;25(5):376-385.

572. Hugel H, Ellershaw JE, Dickman A. Clonazepam as an adjuvant analgesic in patients with cancer-related neuropathic pain. *J Pain Symptom Manage.* 2003;26(6):1073-1074.

573. Tremont-Lukats IW, Challapalli V, McNicol ED, Lau J, Carr DB. Systemic administration of local anesthetics to relieve neuropathic pain: a systematic review and meta-analysis. *Anesth Analg.* 2005;101(6):1738-1749.

574. Challapalli V, Tremont-Lukats IW, McNicol ED, Lau J, Carr DB. Systemic administration of local anesthetic agents to relieve neuropathic pain. *Cochrane Database Syst Rev.* 2005(4):CD003345.

575. Dworkin RH, O'Connor AB, Audette J, et al. Recommendations for the pharmacological management of neuropathic pain: an overview and literature update. *Mayo Clin Proc.* 2010;85(3 Suppl):S3-14.

576. Bell R, Eccleston C, Kalso E. Ketamine as an adjuvant to opioids for cancer pain. *Cochrane Database Syst Rev.* 2003(1):CD003351.

577. Ben-Ari A, Lewis MC, Davidson E. Chronic administration of ketamine for analgesia. *J Pain Palliat Care Pharmacother.* 2007;21(1):7-14.

578. Chizh BA, Headley PM. NMDA antagonists and neuropathic pain—multiple drug targets and multiple uses. *Curr Pharm Des.* 2005;11(23):2977-2994.

579. Yomiya K, Matsuo N, Tomiyasu S, et al. Baclofen as an adjuvant analgesic for cancer pain. *Am J Hosp Palliat Care.* 2009;26(2):112-118.

580. Mercadante S, Casuccio A, Agnello A, Pumo S, Kargar J, Garofalo S. Analgesic effects of nonsteroidal anti-inflammatory drugs in cancer pain due to somatic or visceral mechanisms. *J Pain Symptom Manage.* 1999;17(5):351-356.

581. Minotti V, De Angelis V, Righetti E, et al. Double-blind evaluation of short-term analgesic efficacy of orally administered diclofenac, diclofenac plus codeine, and diclofenac plus imipramine in chronic cancer pain. *Pain.* 1998;74(2-3):133-137.

582. Kenner DJ, Bhagat S, Fullerton SL. Daily subcutaneous parecoxib injection for cancer pain: an open label pilot study. *J Palliat Med.* 2015;18(4):366-372.

583. Stambaugh JE, Jr., Drew J. The combination of ibuprofen and oxycodone/acetaminophen in the management of chronic cancer pain. *Clin Pharmacol Ther.* 1988;44(6):665-669.

584. Myers KG, Trotman IF. Use of ketorolac by continuous subcutaneous infusion for the control of cancer-related pain. *Postgrad Med J.* 1994;70(823):359-362.

585. Porta-Sales J, Garzon-Rodriguez C, Llorens-Torrome S, Brunelli C, Pigni A, Caraceni A. Evidence on the analgesic role of bisphosphonates and denosumab in the treatment of pain due to bone metastases: a systematic review within the European Association for Palliative Care guidelines project. *Palliat Med.* 2017;31(1):5-25.

586. Costa L, Major PP. Effect of bisphosphonates on pain and quality of life in patients with bone metastases. *Nat Clin Pract Oncol.* 2009;6(3):163-174.

587. Miksad RA, Lai KC, Dodson TB, et al. Quality of life implications of bisphosphonate-associated osteonecrosis of the jaw. *Oncologist.* 2011;16(1):121-132.

588. Park-Wyllie LY, Mamdani MM, Juurlink DN, et al. Bisphosphonate use and the risk of subtrochanteric or femoral shaft fractures in older women. *JAMA.* 2011;305(8):783-789.

589. Van Poznak CH, Temin S, Yee GC, et al. American Society of Clinical Oncology executive summary of the clinical practice guideline update on the role of bone-modifying agents in metastatic breast cancer. *J Clin Oncol.* 2011;29(9):1221-1227.

590. Smith MR, Coleman RE, Klotz L, et al. Denosumab for the prevention of skeletal complications in metastatic castration-resistant prostate cancer: comparison of skeletal-related events and symptomatic skeletal events. *Ann Oncol.* 2015;26(2):368-374.

591. Diel IJ, Body JJ, Stopeck AT, et al. The role of denosumab in the prevention of hypercalcaemia of malignancy in cancer patients with metastatic bone disease. *Eur J Cancer.* 2015;51(11):1467-1475.

592. Gnant M, Pfeiler G, Dubsky PC, et al. Adjuvant denosumab in breast cancer (ABCSG-18): a multicentre, randomised, double-blind, placebo-controlled trial. *Lancet.* 2015;386(9992):433-443.

593. Hendriks LE, Hermans BC, van den Beuken-van Everdingen MH, Hochstenbag MM, Dingemans AM. Effect of bisphosphonates, denosumab, and radioisotopes on bone pain and quality of life in patients with non-small cell lung cancer and bone metastases: a systematic review. *J Thorac Oncol.* 2016;11(2):155-173.

594. Stopeck AT, Fizazi K, Body JJ, et al. Erratum to: Safety of long-term denosumab therapy: results from the open label extension phase of two phase 3 studies in patients with metastatic breast and prostate cancer. *Support Care Cancer.* 2015.

595. Autio KA, Farooki A, Glezerman IG, et al. Severe hypocalcemia associated with denosumab in metastatic castration-resistant prostate cancer: risk factors and precautions for treating physicians. *Clin Genitourin Cancer.* 2015;13(4):e305-309.

596. Martinez-Zapata MJ, Roque M, Alonso-Coello P, Catala E. Calcitonin for metastatic bone pain. *Cochrane Database Syst Rev.* 2006;3:CD003223.

597. Resmini G, Ratti C, Canton G, Murena L, Moretti A, Iolascon G. Treatment of complex regional pain syndrome. *Clin Cases Miner Bone Metab.* 2015;12(Suppl 1):26-30.

598. Wertli MM, Kessels AG, Perez RS, Bachmann LM, Brunner F. Rational pain management in complex regional pain syndrome 1 (CRPS 1)—a network meta-analysis. *Pain Med.* 2014;15(9):1575-1589.

599. Maihofner C, Seifert F, Markovic K. Complex regional pain syndromes: new pathophysiological concepts and therapies. *Eur J Neurol.* 2010;17(5):649-660.

600. Christensen MH, Petersen LJ. Radionuclide treatment of painful bone metastases in patients with breast cancer: a systematic review. *Cancer Treat Res.* 2012;38(2):164-171.

601. Cheng A, Chen S, Zhang Y, Yin D, Dong M. The tolerance and therapeutic efficacy of rhenium-188 hydroxyethylidene diphosphonate in advanced cancer patients with painful osseous metastases. *Cancer Biother Radiopharm*. 2011;26(2):237-244.

602. Roque IFM, Martinez-Zapata MJ, Scott-Brown M, Alonso-Coello P. Radioisotopes for metastatic bone pain. *Cochrane Database Syst Rev*. 2011(7):CD003347.

603. Frech EJ, Adler DG. Endoscopic therapy for malignant bowel obstruction. *J Support Oncol*. 2007;5(7):303-310, 319.

604. Kucukmetin A, Naik R, Galaal K, Bryant A, Dickinson HO. Palliative surgery versus medical management for bowel obstruction in ovarian cancer. *Cochrane Database Syst Rev*. 2010(7):CD007792.

605. Laval G, Girardier J, Lassauniere JM, Leduc B, Haond C, Schaerer R. The use of steroids in the management of inoperable intestinal obstruction in terminal cancer patients: do they remove the obstruction? *Palliat Med*. 2000;14(1):3-10.

606. Feuer DJ, Broadley KE. Systematic review and meta-analysis of corticosteroids for the resolution of malignant bowel obstruction in advanced gynaecological and gastrointestinal cancers. Systematic Review Steering Committee. *Ann Oncol*. 1999;10(9):1035-1041.

607. Davis MP, Furste A. Glycopyrrolate: a useful drug in the palliation of mechanical bowel obstruction. *J Pain Symptom Manage*. 1999;18(3):153-154.

608. Dean A. The palliative effects of octreotide in cancer patients. *Chemotherapy*. 2001;47 Suppl 2:54-61.

609. Ripamonti C, Mercadante S, Groff L, Zecca E, De Conno F, Casuccio A. Role of octreotide, scopolamine butylbromide, and hydration in symptom control of patients with inoperable bowel obstruction and nasogastric tubes: a prospective randomized trial. *J Pain Symptom Manage*. 2000;19(1):23-34.

610. Mercadante S, Ripamonti C, Casuccio A, Zecca E, Groff L. Comparison of octreotide and hyoscine butylbromide in controlling gastrointestinal symptoms due to malignant inoperable bowel obstruction. *Support Care Cancer*. 2000;8(3):188-191.

611. Mystakidou K, Tsilika E, Kalaidopoulou O, Chondros K, Georgaki S, Papadimitriou L. Comparison of octreotide administration vs conservative treatment in the management of inoperable bowel obstruction in patients with far advanced cancer: a randomized, double-blind, controlled clinical trial. *Anticancer Res*. 2002;22(2B):1187-1192.

612. Murphy E, Prommer EE, Mihalyo M, Wilcock A. Octreotide. *J Pain Symptom Manage*. 2010;40(1):142-148.

613. Blaes AH, Kreitzer MJ, Torkelson C, Haddad T. Nonpharmacologic complementary therapies in symptom management for breast cancer survivors. *Semin Oncol*. 2011;38(3):394-402.

614. Brogan S, Junkins S. Interventional therapies for the management of cancer pain. *J Support Oncol*. 8(2):52-59.

615. Arcidiacono PG, Calori G, Carrara S, McNicol ED, Testoni PA. Celiac plexus block for pancreatic cancer pain in adults. *Cochrane Database Syst Rev*. 2011(3):CD007519.

616. Kaufman M, Singh G, Das S, et al. Efficacy of endoscopic ultrasound-guided celiac plexus block and celiac plexus neurolysis for managing abdominal pain associated with chronic pancreatitis and pancreatic cancer. *J Clin Gastroenterol*. 2010;44(2):127-134.

617. Carnes D, Homer KE, Miles CL, et al. Effective delivery styles and content for self-management interventions for chronic musculoskeletal pain: a systematic literature review. *Clin J Pain*. 2012;28(4):344-354.

618. Kwekkeboom KL, Cherwin CH, Lee JW, Wanta B. Mind-body treatments for the pain-fatigue-sleep disturbance symptom cluster in persons with cancer. *J Pain Symptom Manage*. 2010;39(1):126-138.

619. Bardia A, Barton DL, Prokop LJ, Bauer BA, Moynihan TJ. Efficacy of complementary and alternative medicine therapies in relieving cancer pain: a systematic review. *J Clin Oncol*. 2006;24(34):5457-5464.

620. Bradt J, Dileo C, Grocke D, Magill L. Music interventions for improving psychological and physical outcomes in cancer patients. *Cochrane Database Syst Rev*. 2011(8):CD006911.

621. Bradt J, Goodill SW, Dileo C. Dance/movement therapy for improving psychological and physical outcomes in cancer patients. *Cochrane Database Syst Rev.* 2011(10):CD007103.

622. Srbely JZ, Dickey JP. Randomized controlled study of the antinociceptive effect of ultrasound on trigger point sensitivity: novel applications in myofascial therapy? *Clin Rehabil.* 2007;21(5):411-417.

623. Moreno MA, Furtner F, Rivara FP. How parents can help children cope with procedures and pain. *Arch Pediatr Adolesc Med.* 2011;165(9):872.

624. Accardi MC, Milling LS. The effectiveness of hypnosis for reducing procedure-related pain in children and adolescents: a comprehensive methodological review. *J Behav Med.* 2009;32(4):328-339.

625. American Academy of Pediatrics, American Academy of Pediatric Dentistry. Guideline for monitoring and management of pediatric patients during and after sedation for diagnostic and therapeutic procedures. *Pediatric Dent.* 2008;30(7 Suppl):143-159.

626. Cheshire WP. Fosphenytoin: an intravenous option for the management of acute trigeminal neuralgia crisis. *J Pain Symptom Manage.* 2001;21(6):506-510.

627. Meals CG, Mullican BD, Shaffer CM, Dangerfield PF, Ramirez RP. Ketamine infusion for sickle cell crisis pain in an adult. *J Pain Symptom Manage.* 2011;42(3):e7-9.

628. McHardy P, McDonnell C, Lorenzo AJ, Salle JL, Campbell FA. Management of priapism in a child with sickle cell anemia; successful outcome using epidural analgesia. *Can J Anaesth.* 2007;54(8):642-645.

629. Levy MH, Back A, Benedetti C, et al. NCCN clinical practice guidelines in oncology: palliative care. *J Natl Compr Canc Netw.* 2009;7(4):436-473.

630. Twycross RG, Fairfield S. Pain in far-advanced cancer. *Pain.* 1982;14(3):303-310.

631. Goudas LC, Bloch R, Gialeli-Goudas M, Lau J, Carr DB. The epidemiology of cancer pain. *Cancer Invest.* 2005;23(2):182-190.

632. Grond S, Zech D, Lynch J, Diefenbach C, Schug SA, Lehmann KA. Validation of World Health Organization guidelines for pain relief in head and neck cancer. A prospective study. *Ann Otol Rhinol Laryngol.* 1993;102(5):342-348.

633. Trevino CM, deRoon-Cassini T, Brasel K. Does opiate use in traumatically injured individuals worsen pain and psychological outcomes? *J Pain.* 2013;14(4):424-430.

634. Imani F, Motavaf M, Safari S, Alavian SM. The therapeutic use of analgesics in patients with liver cirrhosis: a literature review and evidence-based recommendations. *Hepat Mon.* 2014;14(10):e23539.

635. Delco F, Tchambaz L, Schlienger R, Drewe J, Krahenbuhl S. Dose adjustment in patients with liver disease. *Drug Saf.* 2005;28(6):529-545.

636. Arnman R, Olsson R. Elimination of paracetamol in chronic liver disease. *Acta Hepatogastroenterol (Stuttg).* 1978;25(4):283-286.

637. Andreasen PB, Hutters L. Paracetamol (acetaminophen) clearance in patients with cirrhosis of the liver. *Acta Med Scand Suppl.* 1979;624:99-105.

638. Benson GD, Koff RS, Tolman KG. The therapeutic use of acetaminophen in patients with liver disease. *Am J Ther.* 2005;12(2):133-141.

639. Heard K, Green JL, Bailey JE, Bogdan GM, Dart RC. A randomized trial to determine the change in alanine aminotransferase during 10 days of paracetamol (acetaminophen) administration in subjects who consume moderate amounts of alcohol. *Aliment Pharmacol Ther.* 2007;26(2):283-290.

640. Kuffner EK, Green JL, Bogdan GM, et al. The effect of acetaminophen (four grams a day for three consecutive days) on hepatic tests in alcoholic patients—a multicenter randomized study. *BMC Med.* 2007;5:13.

641. Chandok N, Watt KD. Pain management in the cirrhotic patient: the clinical challenge. *Mayo Clin Proc.* 2010;85(5):451-458.

642. Claria J, Kent JD, Lopez-Parra M, et al. Effects of celecoxib and naproxen on renal function in nonazotemic patients with cirrhosis and ascites. *Hepatology.* 2005;41(3):579-587.

643. Harris RC, Breyer MD. Update on cyclooxygenase-2 inhibitors. *Clin J Am Soc Nephrol.* 2006;1(2):236-245.

644. Hasselstrom J, Eriksson S, Persson A, Rane A, Svensson JO, Sawe J. The metabolism and bioavailability of morphine in patients with severe liver cirrhosis. *Br J Clin Pharmacol.* 1990;29(3):289-297.

645. Durnin C, Hind ID, Ghani SP, Yates DB, Molz KH. Pharmacokinetics of oral immediate-release hydromorphone (Dilaudid IR) in subjects with moderate hepatic impairment. *Proc West Pharmacol Soc.* 2001;44:83-84.

646. Hutchinson MR, Menelaou A, Foster DJ, Coller JK, Somogyi AA. CYP2D6 and CYP3A4 involvement in the primary oxidative metabolism of hydrocodone by human liver microsomes. *Br J Clin Pharmacol.* 2004;57(3):287-297.

647. Chen H, Shen ZY, Xu W, et al. Expression of P450 and nuclear receptors in normal and end-stage Chinese livers. *World J Gastroenterol.* 2014;20(26):8681-8690.

648. Tallgren M, Olkkola KT, Seppala T, Hockerstedt K, Lindgren L. Pharmacokinetics and ventilatory effects of oxycodone before and after liver transplantation. *Clin Pharmacol Ther.* 1997;61(6):655-661.

649. Hoyumpa AM, Schenker S. Is glucuronidation truly preserved in patients with liver disease? *Hepatology.* 1991;13(4):786-795.

650. Debinski HS, Lee CS, Danks JA, Mackenzie PI, Desmond PV. Localization of uridine 5'-diphosphate-glucuronosyltransferase in human liver injury. *Gastroenterology.* 1995;108(5):1464-1469.

651. Iribarne C, Picart D, Dreano Y, Bail JP, Berthou F. Involvement of cytochrome P450 3A4 in N-dealkylation of buprenorphine in human liver microsomes. *Life Sci.* 1997;60(22):1953-1964.

652. Poder U, Ljungman G, von Essen L. Parents' perceptions of their children's cancer-related symptoms during treatment: a prospective, longitudinal study. *J Pain Symptom Manage.* 2010;40(5):661-670.

653. Po C, Benini F, Sainati L, Farina MI, Cesaro S, Agosto C. The management of procedural pain at the Italian Centers of Pediatric Hematology-Oncology: state-of-the-art and future directions. *Support Care Cancer.* 2011.

654. Lundeberg T, Lund I, Dahlin L, et al. Reliability and responsiveness of three different pain assessments. *J Rehabil Med.* 2001;33(6):279-283.

655. Mercadante S, Aielli F, Masedu F, et al. Pattern of symptoms and symptomatic treatment in adults and the aged population: a retrospective analysis of advanced cancer patients followed at home. *Curr Med Res Opin.* 2016;32(5):893-898.

656. Mercadante S, Aielli F, Masedu F, Valenti M, Verna L, Porzio G. Age differences in the last week of life in advanced cancer patients followed at home. *Support Care Cancer.* 2016;24(4):1889-1895.

657. Shega JW, Dale W, Andrew M, Paice J, Rockwood K, Weiner DK. Persistent pain and frailty: a case for homeostenosis. *J Am Geriatr Soc.* 2012;60(1):113-117.

658. Mercadante S, Aielli F, Masedu F, Valenti M, Ficorella C, Porzio G. Pain characteristics and analgesic treatment in an aged adult population: a 4-week retrospective analysis of advanced cancer patients followed at home. *Drugs Aging.* 2015;32(4):315-320.

659. Ashby M, Fleming B, Wood M, Somogyi A. Plasma morphine and glucuronide (M3G and M6G) concentrations in hospice inpatients. *J Pain Symptom Manage.* 1997;14(3):157-167.

660. Sorkin BA, Rudy TE, Hanlon RB, Turk DC, Stieg RL. Chronic pain in old and young patients: differences appear less important than similarities. *J Gerontol.* 1990;45(2):P64-68.

661. Vigano A, Bruera E, Suarez-Almazor ME. Age, pain intensity, and opioid dose in patients with advanced cancer. *Cancer.* 1998;83(6):1244-1250.

662. Hall S, Gallagher RM, Gracely E, Knowlton C, Wescules D. The terminal cancer patient: effects of age, gender, and primary tumor site on opioid dose. *Pain Med.* 2003;4(2):125-134.

663. Mercadante S, Arcuri E. Pharmacological management of cancer pain in the elderly. *Drugs Aging.* 2007;24(9):761-776.

664. Wong NA, Jones HW. An analysis of discharge drug prescribing amongst elderly patients with renal impairment. *Postgrad Med J.* 1998;74(873):420-422.

665. Pereira J, Hanson J, Bruera E. The frequency and clinical course of cognitive impairment in patients with terminal cancer. *Cancer.* 1997;79(4):835-842.

666. Schmader KE, Baron R, Haanpaa ML, et al. Treatment considerations for elderly and frail patients with neuropathic pain. *Mayo Clin Proc.* 2010;85(3 Suppl):S26-32.

667. McLachlan AJ, Bath S, Naganathan V, et al. Clinical pharmacology of analgesic medicines in older people: impact of frailty and cognitive impairment. *Br J Clin Pharmacol.* 2011;71(3):351-364.

668. American Geriatrics Society Beers Criteria Update Expert Panel. American Geriatrics Society updated Beers Criteria for potentially inappropriate medication use in older adults. *J Am Geriatr Soc.* 2012;60(4):616-631.

669. Griebling TL. Re: American Geriatrics Society 2015 updated Beers Criteria for Potentially Inappropriate Medication Use in Older Adults. *J Urol.* 2016;195(3):667-669.

670. American Geriatrics Society Panel on Pharmacological Management of Persistent Pain in Older Persons. Pharmacological management of persistent pain in older persons. *J Am Geriatr Soc.* 2009;57(8):1331-1346.

671. van Ojik AL, Jansen PA, Brouwers JR, van Roon EN. Treatment of chronic pain in older people: evidence-based choice of strong-acting opioids. *Drugs Aging.* 2012;29(8):615-625.

672. Lee J, Lakha SF, Mailis A. Efficacy of low-dose oral liquid morphine for elderly patients with chronic non-cancer pain: retrospective chart review. *Drugs Real World Outcomes.* 2015;2(4):369-376.

673. Gianni W, Madaio AR, Ceci M, et al. Transdermal buprenorphine for the treatment of chronic noncancer pain in the oldest old. *J Pain Symptom Manage.* 2011;41(4):707-714.

674. Yu SY, Sun Y, Zhang HC, et al. Transdermal fentanyl for the management of cancer pain: a survey of 1,664 elderly patients. *Zhonghua Yi Xue Za Zhi.* 2003;83(22):1931-1935.

675. Biondi DM, Xiang J, Etropolski M, Moskovitz B. Tolerability and efficacy of tapentadol extended release in elderly patients ≥ 75 years of age with chronic osteoarthritis knee or low back pain. *J Opioid Manag.* 2015;11(5):393-403.

676. Guerriero F, Roberto A, Greco MT, Sgarlata C, Rollone M, Corli O. Long-term efficacy and safety of oxycodone-naloxone prolonged release in geriatric patients with moderate-to-severe chronic noncancer pain: a 52-week open-label extension phase study. *Drug Des Devel Ther.* 2016;10:1515-1523.

677. Pergolizzi J, Boger RH, Budd K, et al. Opioids and the management of chronic severe pain in the elderly: consensus statement of an International Expert Panel with focus on the six clinically most often used World Health Organization Step III opioids (buprenorphine, fentanyl, hydromorphone, methadone, morphine, oxycodone). *Pain Pract.* 2008;8(4):287-313.

678. Pergolizzi J, Aloisi AM, Dahan A, et al. Current knowledge of buprenorphine and its unique pharmacological profile. *Pain Pract.* 2010;10(5):428-450.

679. Hirst A, Knight C, Hirst M, Dunlop W, Akehurst R. Tramadol and the risk of fracture in an elderly female population: a cost utility assessment with comparison to transdermal buprenorphine. *Eur J Health Econ.* 2016;17(2):217-227.

680. Turnheim K. Drug therapy in the elderly. *Exp Gerontol.* 2004;39(11-12):1731-1738.

681. Kloke M, Rapp M, Bosse B, Kloke O. Toxicity and/or insufficient analgesia by opioid therapy: risk factors and the impact of changing the opioid. A retrospective analysis of 273 patients observed at a single center. *Support Care Cancer.* 2000;8(6):479-486.

682. Shinde S, Gordon P, Sharma P, Gross J, Davis MP. Use of non-opioid analgesics as adjuvants to opioid analgesia for cancer pain management in an inpatient palliative unit: does this improve pain control and reduce opioid requirements? *Support Care Cancer*. 2015;23(3):695-703.

683. Malec M, Shega JW. Pain management in the elderly. *Med Clin North Am*. 2015;99(2):337-350.

684. Sikka P, Kaushik S, Kumar G, Kapoor S, Bindra VK, Saxena KK. Study of antinociceptive activity of SSRI (fluoxetine and escitalopram) and atypical antidepressants (venlafaxine and mirtazepine) and their interaction with morphine and naloxone in mice. *J Pharm Bioallied Sci*. 2011;3(3):412-416.

685. Ailawadhi S, Sung KW, Carlson LA, Baer MR. Serotonin syndrome caused by interaction between citalopram and fentanyl. *J Clin Pharm Ther*. 2007;32(2):199-202.

686. Schenk M, Wirz S. Serotonin syndrome and pain medication: what is relevant for practice? *Schmerz*. 2015;29(2):229-251.

687. Hillman AD, Witenko CJ, Sultan SM, Gala G. Serotonin syndrome caused by fentanyl and methadone in a burn injury. *Pharmacotherapy*. 2015;35(1):112-117.

688. Dolder C, Nelson M, Stump A. Pharmacological and clinical profile of newer antidepressants: implications for the treatment of elderly patients. *Drugs Aging*. 2010;27(8):625-640.

689. Oakes TM, Katona C, Liu P, Robinson M, Raskin J, Greist JH. Safety and tolerability of duloxetine in elderly patients with major depressive disorder: a pooled analysis of two placebo-controlled studies. *Int Clin Psychopharmacol*. 2013;28(1):1-11.

690. Callegari C, Ielmini M, Bianchi L, Lucano M, Vender S. Antiepileptic drug use in a nursing home setting: a retrospective study in older adults. *Funct Neurol*. 2015:1-7.

691. Herr K, Bjoro K, Decker S. Tools for assessment of pain in nonverbal older adults with dementia: a state-of-the-science review. *J Pain Symptom Manage*. 2006;31(2):170-192.

692. Gibson SJ. What does an increased prevalence of behavioral and psychological symptoms of dementia in individuals with pain mean? *Pain*. 2012;153(2):261-262.

693. Kovach CR, Weissman DE, Griffie J, Matson S, Muchka S. Assessment and treatment of discomfort for people with late-stage dementia. *J Pain Symptom Manage*. 1999;18(6):412-419.

694. Hurley AC, Volicer BJ, Hanrahan PA, Houde S, Volicer L. Assessment of discomfort in advanced Alzheimer patients. *Res Nurs Health*. 1992;15(5):369-377.

695. Warden V, Hurley AC, Volicer L. Development and psychometric evaluation of the Pain Assessment in Advanced Dementia (PAINAD) scale. *J Am Med Dir Assoc*. 2003;4(1):9-15.

696. Feldt KS. The checklist of nonverbal pain indicators (CNPI). *Pain Manag Nurs*. 2000;1(1):13-21.

697. Institute of Medicine. Relieving Pain in America: A Blueprint for Transforming Prevention, Care, Education, and Research. Washington, DC: National Academies Press; 2011. https://www.nap.edu/read/13172/chapter/1. Accessed July 15, 2017.

698. Chen CH, Tang ST, Chen CH. Meta-analysis of cultural differences in Western and Asian patient-perceived barriers to managing cancer pain. *Palliat Med*. 2012;26(3):206-221.

699. Meghani SH, Byun E, Gallagher RM. Time to take stock: a meta-analysis and systematic review of analgesic treatment disparities for pain in the United States. *Pain Med*. 2012;13(2):150-174.

700. Green CR, Anderson KO, Baker TA, et al. The unequal burden of pain: confronting racial and ethnic disparities in pain. *Pain Med*. 2003;4(3):277-294.

701. Ozkan S, Ozkan M, Armay Z. Cultural meaning of cancer suffering. *J Pediatr Hematol Oncol*. 2011;33 Suppl 2:S102-104.

702. Magnusson JE, Fennell JA. Understanding the role of culture in pain: Maori practitioner perspectives relating to the experience of pain. *N Z Med J*. 2011;124(1328):41-51.

703. Delgado-Guay MO, Hui D, Parsons HA, et al. Spirituality, religiosity, and spiritual pain in advanced cancer patients. *J Pain Symptom Manage.* 2011;41(6):986-994.

704. Wein S. Impact of culture on the expression of pain and suffering. *J Pediatr Hematol Oncol.* 2011;33 Suppl 2:S105-107.

705. Armstrong K, Putt M, Halbert CH, et al. Prior experiences of racial discrimination and racial differences in health care system distrust. *Med Care.* 2013;51(2):144-150.

# Index

dantrolene for myoclonus, 70
deafferentiation, 13
deaths, opioid-related, 5
dehydration, hypotension and, 71–72
dehydroepiandrosterone (DHEA), 67
delirium, opioid-induced, 70
delta (DOR) opioid receptors, 31
dementia, 113
denosumab, 10, 96–97
depression, opioids and, 5
desipramine, 87t, 90, 113
desvenlafaxine, 90
dexamethasone, 87t, 100
dexmedetomidine, 91
dextromethorphan, 96
diabetic neuropathy, 32
diazepam, methadone levels and, 43t
diclofenac, 83t, 87t, 93
diflunisal, 82t
divalproex, 88t
docetaxel, 13
dosages, misconceptions, 79
doxepin, 48, 87t, 93
drug-drug interactions in older adults, 111
dry mouth, opioids and, 61
duloxetine, 87t, 90, 113
Duragesic, 39
dynorphin, expression of, 11
dysesthesia, 11

Edmonton Symptom Assessment Scale (ESAS), 18
electrophysiological tests, 25t
emesis, opioid-induced, 65
emetogenic reflexes, 65
end-of-dose-failure pain, 21
end-of-life care, 27–32
endocrinopathies, opioid-induced, 67–68
epidural administration, 51, 52
episodic pain, 50
equianalgesic conversion data, 36–39
escape doses, 44
estradiol levels, 68
estrogen deficiencies, 67

etodolac, 85t
European Association for Palliative Care, 105

Faces Pain Scale (FPS), 19f
falls, opioids and, 5
family education, adherence to plans and, 103
fatigue, opioids and, 67
fecal retention in older adults, 112
fentanyl. see also transdermal fentanyl (TDF); Transmucosal Immediate Release Fentanyl (TIRF)
      considerations, 39–44
      delirium and, 70
      epidural-sequestered, 52
      equianalgesic doses, 34t
      formulations, 47
      mechanism of action, 40
      metabolism of, 109
      in older adults, 113
      parenteral to transdermal conversion, 47
      QTc prolongation and, 62
      rapid-onset formulations, 45, 58
      starting intrathecal doses, 53t
      transdermal, 39–41, 110
fibromyalgia, 7, 32
fluoroquinolones, methadone levels and, 43t
flurbiprofen, 83t
Food and Drug Administration (FDA), 33
frailty, pain and, 111

GABA agonists, 88t
gabapentin
      adjuvant use of, 88t
      mechanism of action, 94–95
      for myoclonus, 70
      for neuropathic pain, 10, 94–95
      in older adults, 113
      topical use of, 94
gabapentinoids
      in liver disease, 110
      mechanisms of action, 94–95
      for neuropathic pain, 94–95
      in older adults, 113
galactorrhea, 67

lidocaine
- for acute pain crises, 100
- adjuvant use of, 87t, 88t
- analgesic use of, 93
- local anesthetic, 53

Likert scale, 110

lipophilicity, drug administration and, 47, 48

liver disease, people with, 105–110

liver hypoxia, analgesic use in, 105

local anesthetics, side effects of, 53

lymphedema, pain of, 86

macrolides, methadone levels and, 43t

McGill Pain Questionnaire (MPQ), 18

meclofenamic acid, 84t

memantine, 89t, 96

meperidine, 33, 35t

metabolic abnormalities in older adults, 112

metabolic syndrome, opioids and, 67

metastatic disease, pain and, 8, 106t

methadone, 41–42
- considerations, 39–44
- cortisol levels and, 68
- equianalgesic doses, 35t
- half-life of, 36, 41
- metabolism of, 41, 109
- morphine conversion to, 43t
- in older adults, 112, 113
- oral bioavailability of, 41
- patient compliance, 43t
- PEG delivery, 51
- potency of, 62
- QTc prolongation and, 62
- risks associated with, 41
- rotation of, 42
- safe dosing, 42–44
- subcutaneous, 49
- sublingual, 45

methylphenidate, 69

metoclopramide, 66

mexiletine, 88t

milnacipran, 90

Model for End-stage Liver Disease scores, 105

mood changes, opioids and, 67

mood disorders, opioids and, 69

morphine
- for acute pain crises, 100
- conversion to methadone, 43t
- conversion to TDF, 40t
- delirium and, 70
- epidural analgesia, 52–53
- equianalgesic doses, 34t
- immunosuppression and, 68–69
- infusion, 49
- intrathecal analgesia, 52–53
- osteoporosis and, 66
- PEG delivery, 51
- rectal administration, 48
- release, 33
- rescue doses, 44
- respiratory depression and, 71–72
- starting intrathecal doses, 53t
- transdermal fentanyl and, 39–41
- WHO analgesic ladder, 36

morphine sulfate (Embeda, Kadian), 51

mu-agonist opioids, 31, 33, 36

mu (MOR) opioid receptors, 31, 71

musculoskeletal examination, 24t

musculoskeletal system, opioid-related adverse events, 66

myelography in pain, 25t

myoclonus, opioids and, 69–70

N-methyl-D-aspartate (NMDA)
- inhibitors, 89t
- receptors, 41
- subunits, 11, 32

nabilone, 87t

nabiximol, 92–93

nabumetone, 85t

naloxone, 33, 63

naproxen, 48, 83t

National Comprehensive Cancer Network, 105

nausea and vomiting, 65–66

nerve block, diagnostic, 25t

nerve damage, 13

radiation therapy, pain related to, 108t

radionucleotides, bone-seeking, 97–98

radiopharmaceuticals, 89t

rapid eye movement (REM), 71

receptor activator of nuclear factor kappa B-receptor (RANK), 10

receptor activator of nuclear factor kappa B-receptor ligand (RANK-L), 10

rectal administration, 48

relaxation training, 99

renal failure, opioid selection in, 36

rescue doses, 44, 49–50

respiratory depression
  life-threatening, 71–72
  opioids and, 61
  risk with TDF, 39
  spinal anesthesia and, 51–52

rhenium-188, 97

rhenium-223, 97

rifampin, methadone levels and, 43t

Risk Evaluation and Mitigation Strategy (REMS) Access program, 40

risk management, 72–79

risperidone, 66

ropivacaine, 53

rostral cingulate cortex, 8

rostral ventromedial medulla (RVM), 8, 9f

routes of administration, 45–57
  misconceptions, 79

salicylates, 82t

samarium-153, 89t, 97

sarcopenia, 5

scopolamine, 66, 89t, 98

sedatives, contraindications, 110

selective serotonin reuptake inhibitors (SSRIs), 43t

Self-Reported Leeds Assessment of Neuropathic Symptoms and Signs Scale, 8

senna regimen, 64t

serotonin-norepinephrine reuptake inhibitors (SNRIs), 87t, 90

sexual dysfunction, opioids and, 61, 67

sigma-1 receptor blockage, 31

skin changes, 13

sleep-disordered breathing, 5, 42, 61, 70–71

sodium channel blockers, 88t

sodium channels, 10

soft tissue pain, tumor-related, 106t

somatic pain, 13

somatostatin analogues, 89t

somnolence, opioids and, 69

sorbitol regimen, 64t

spinal analgesic therapy, 51

spinal cord, bone pain and, 11

spinal extracellular fluid, morphine in, 52

spinal opioid pharmacology, 52–53

St. John's Wort, 43t

strontium-89, 89t, 97

subarachnoid administration, 51

subcutaneous administration, 45, 49

sublingual administration, 45, 47, 48

substance P, 10, 31

substance use disorders, 77

sufentanil, 52, 53t

suffering, pain-related, 5

suicidal ideation, 69

sulindac, 84t

suppositories, 48

surgery, pain related to, 108t

sweating, abnormal, 13

tanezumab, 10–11

tapentadol
  abuse-deterrent technology, 33
  adverse effects of, 33
  equianalgesic doses, 35t
  extended-release, 112
  mechanisms of action, 33

testosterone levels, 62, 67

testosterone replacement therapy, 68

thalidomide, 13

THC, adjuvant use of, 87t

therapeutic massage, 99

tizanidine, 87t, 91

tolerance, 77–78

tolmetin, 84t